1997

Contracting with
Managed C
Organizatio

A Guide for the Health Care Provider

Joseph A. Welfeld, FACHE

AHA books are published by American Hospital Publishing, Inc.,
an American Hospital Association company

This publication is designed to provide accurate and authoritative information in regard to the subject matter covered. It is sold with the understanding that neither the author nor the publisher is engaged in rendering legal, accounting, or other professional service. If legal advice or other expert assistance is required, the services of a competent professional person should be sought.

The views expressed in this publication are strictly those of the author and do not necessarily represent official positions of the American Hospital Association.

Library of Congress Cataloging-in-Publication Data

Welfeld, Joseph A.
    Contracting with managed care organizations : a guide for the health care provider / Joseph A. Welfeld.
        p.   cm.
    ISBN 1-55648-156-X
    1. Hospitals—United States—Business management. 2. Hospital care—Contracting out—United States. 3. Managed care plans (Medical care)—United States. I. Title.
    [DNLM: 1. Managed Care Programs—United States. 2. Contract Services. 3. Hospital Administration—United States.   W 130 AA1 W445c 1996]
    RA971.3.W455   1996
    362.1'1'068—dc20
    DNLM/DLC
    for Library of Congress   96–12508
                                                                                  CIP

Catalog no. 131003

©1996 by American Hospital Publishing, Inc.,
an American Hospital Association company

Printed in the USA

AHA is a service mark of the American Hospital Association used under license by American Hospital Publishing, Inc.

Text set in Trump Medieval
4M—05/96—0436

Richard Hill, Senior Editor
Lee Benaka, Editor
Peggy DuMais, Assistant Manager, Production
Marcia Bottoms, Books Division Director

This book is dedicated to Blossom, Robyn, and Michael. I thank you for patiently accompanying me on my travels up, down, up and around, on the roller coaster called managed care.

Contents

About the Author

Joseph A. Welfeld, FACHE, has worked in the health care field for more than 20 years and in managed care for close to 15 years. He is a principal with McManis Associates Inc., a management and research consulting firm based in Washington, D.C. Mr. Welfeld, who is based in the northeast, works with hospitals, hospital networks, physician groups, physician networks, home health care organizations, HMOs, and other managed care organizations.

Mr. Welfeld previously served as regional vice-president for United HealthCare Corporation, one of the largest managed care organizations in the United States, and as founding chief executive officer of Ocean State Physicians Health Plan in Warwick, Rhode Island. During his tenure at Ocean State (now United Health Plans of New England, Inc.), Ocean State was listed as number 2 in the *INC* 500 list of fastest-growing privately held organizations in the United States. (Ocean State was acquired by United HealthCare in 1992.) Mr. Welfeld also served as executive director of Nassau Physicians Review Organization, the PSRO for Long Island; as executive director of the Long Island Cancer Council, a National Cancer Institute model demonstration program; and as assistant director of King County Hospital in Brooklyn.

Mr. Welfeld earned an MBA in health care administration from Baruch College and the Mt. Sinai School of Medicine, both in New York City. He is a fellow in the American College of Health Care Executives, past chairman of the College's Managed Care Executives Committee, and chairman of the Managed Care Committee of the Health Care Financial Management Association's metro New York chapter.

Acknowledgments

A book of this nature represents the documentation of experience gained from managed care contract negotiations during a career on both the HMO and provider sides of the negotiating table. I therefore must thank those who have given me the opportunity to gain this experience, including my employers, and those clients who have permitted me to advise and represent them.

This book would not be possible without the assistance of Richard A. Hill, Senior Editor at American Hospital Publishing, Inc. Rick provided the enthusiasm and constructive criticism to initiate the project and keep it on target.

I would also like to acknowledge the personal and professional support and assistance of Jeffrey Becker of Epstein, Becker, and Green, P.C. Jeff has been a friend and confidant for many years. Without his counseling, encouragement, and support, the opportunity to write this book would never have occurred.

Finally, I must thank my family for patiently supporting my career and this effort.

Introduction

A little more than 10 years ago, the term *managed care* meant relatively little to most hospital and health care executives and was unknown to the general population. Today, managed care might even make David Letterman's top-10 list and is probably the most frequent response offered when health care executives and physicians are asked, "What keeps you up at night?" Similarly and correspondingly, the concept of managed care contracting has grown in stature and now has significant strategic importance in most health care organizations.

This book presents a strategic approach to managed care contracting, from preparing a provider organization for the managed care environment to negotiating contract terms. The book should be viewed as a reference manual to be used as a guide when evaluating and negotiating managed care agreements. It can be used as a reference to assist a hospital in determining strategic managed care relationships. It also can be used as an adjunct to the efforts of a hospital's legal counsel, helping to frame the key issues that might make or break a deal. Finally, this book can be used by hospital managers to help orient employees to the new managed care–dominated world of health care.

Chapter One

Understanding Your Position

A provider organization should begin the process of negotiating managed care contracts by understanding its overall strategic position with regard to managed care. Although this seems obvious, managed care contracting activity often takes place outside the context of the organization's strategic plan and at an organizational level where the long-term strategic vision may not be taken into account. Instead, the managed care office is charged with signing as many contracts as possible, and its performance is measured based on that criterion.

In the frenzy of managed care growth and fear, many providers have approached the contracting process without the intensive analysis it deserves. Given managed care's growing importance in all areas of health care delivery including Medicare, Medicaid, and worker's compensation, it is imperative that the contracting process be approached strategically. This approach includes assessment of your organization's position in the market, honest analysis of the infrastructure available to negotiate and implement managed care agreements, and clear understanding of the stakeholders who must be involved. It also includes identification of the individual who can commit your organization during the negotiation process and an understanding of the terms that the organization will accept in these agreements. Only when these issues are clear can the negotiating team make a reasoned evaluation of a proposed managed care contract.

Understanding Your Strengths and Weaknesses

The process of negotiating managed care contracts requires two significant, perhaps gut-wrenching, assessments. First, providers must objectively assess the strength of the managed care organization (MCO) with which negotiations are being undertaken. Second, and more important, each provider organization must conduct an objective self-assessment in order to understand its relative position in the market, how important this contract is to the overall organizational strategic plan, and the provider's relative strength (or weakness) in the negotiation process.

Generally, as the importance of managed care continues to grow in a geographic region, a level of panic sets in at the provider level, giving the MCO much more negotiation leverage. Most provider organizations have significant value and strength that they fail to take into account during negotiations. Unfortunately, and just as damaging, many are unwilling or unable to face their internal weaknesses and make the changes necessary to improve their leverage position. This often imposes a significant negotiating deficit with MCOs that may have done their homework and know as much (sometimes more) about their negotiation opponents.

An organization's strengths and weaknesses fall into two categories: position in the market and internal infrastructure. Although an organization's marketplace position is important for its strategic positioning and leverage in contract negotiations, its internal infrastructure is critical for both the negotiation and implementation processes. In addition, external market issues that affect an organization's market position may be more difficult to alter as quickly as many infrastructure issues.

External Market Issues

A number of factors that position a provider organization in the market are related to the image it may have created over a number of years. This image includes its perceived quality, the strength of its medical staff, and the appearance of its facilities. Although these "soft" criteria may have been prevalent in early stages of managed care contracting activity, MCOs now use more specific and sophisticated criteria to select their preferred providers. Therefore, your organization should use the following specific criteria (among others) as it undergoes self-assessment to determine the strength of its negotiating position:

- *Competitive cost structure:* Much of the information regarding a hospital's cost structure is available to MCOs through cost reports filed with HCFA and sometimes state agencies.
- *DRG performance indicators*: Managed care organizations are evaluated by large employers using Healthplan Employer Data Information Set (HEDIS) criteria developed by the National Center for Quality Assurance (NCQA). It is imperative, then, that your organization assess its competitive performance for each DRG identified by HEDIS.

- *Alliances/affiliations:* A provider organization's membership in an alliance or larger network can provide additional contract negotiation leverage.
- *Geographic market:* Territorial exclusivity can be a significant negotiating factor. For example, if your hospital is the only player in a key geographic market, the negotiating strategy will differ greatly than if it must go head to head with a competitor on price and quality issues.
- *Physician support for managed care:* Separate and distinct from the issue of joint physician–hospital contracting is the perception of the medical staff's willingness to support managed care initiatives. If your medical staff has not been supportive of managed care in the past, your negotiating position may be more difficult, even if medical staff attitudes have changed.
- *Service delivery network:* The array of health care services provided is a critical market issue. This includes the distribution of primary and specialty physicians as well as the range of services, from ambulatory care to home care.

Internal Infrastructure

Successful negotiation of managed care agreements also requires careful assessment of your organization's infrastructure capabilities to ensure that requirements defined in a contractual agreement can be met. These requirements may range from your negotiating team's ability to be successful to your organization's ability to identify managed care patients and process them appropriately. Of greater importance, however, is your organization's ability to accept financial risk arrangements and/or discounted fees offered by MCOs. Therefore, some important criteria to be used in the self-assessment process include the following:

- *Management staff capabilities:* Organizations and managers successful under the fee-for-service reimbursement methodologies of the past may not have the competencies required for managed care. Being able to accept uncertainty and risk, understanding customer service–driven needs of managed care organizations, and acknowledging the need to manage new relationships with physicians are among these competencies.

   Staff competencies that need to be examined carefully include those of senior managers in finance, medical affairs, patient services, and utilization management. Assessing these capabilities will help determine the types of arrangements that can be accepted, from both an operational and risk perspective. This assessment also will help identify the appropriate negotiating team and the key negotiator.

- *Payer mix:* It is important to understand the array of patients currently serviced by your organization prior to entering a managed care negotiation process. This is because the spectrum of "covered lives" being offered by the MCO may complement, supplement, or even replace your current mix—which could have significant financial, political, and operational implications.

- *Information systems:* Systems that support evaluation and measurement of clinical and financial performance are critical to success. If these systems are not in place, those negotiating and monitoring performance of managed care agreements will be severely hampered. Information system availability and capability also should influence the levels of reimbursement and performance acceptable in an agreement under negotiation.

- *Organizational culture/structure:* Organizations that succeeded under fee for service may have cultures that differ markedly from those that will be successful under managed care. An organizational structure conducive to a culture that focuses on customer service, is less consensus driven, and can react quickly to change is at a negotiations advantage.

- *Commitment to utilization management:* Ongoing measurement of hospital and physician performance is mandatory for success in managed care contracting. Systems must be in place to measure provider performance down to the level of individual physicians by DRG and service category. Although utilization review programs may be in place to meet regulatory requirements, the programs may not have the enforcement teeth required to make economic credentialing decisions stick.

- *Operations efficiency:* Honest assessment of your facility's operating efficiency is critical for both successful fee negotiations and physician–hospital capitated arrangements. Although some reimbursement systems in the past have been case based and/or cost based, and providers were able to operate effectively within their reimbursement parameters, most future managed care agreements will be per diem agreements. This will require optimum operational efficiency from the moment a patient enters the system. In joint physician–hospital contracting (either through physician–hospital organizations [PHOs] or global fee arrangements), physicians will need constant reassurance that the hospital is operating at peak efficiency and, therefore, that the percentage of health care dollars the hospital receives does not eat into the physicians' piece of the pie.

Developing Clear Goals for the Contracting Effort

A managed care contracting strategy must be predicated on a set of clear goals and objectives. Given your hospital's market position—a position honestly evaluated during self-assessment—the hospital should clarify its short- and long-range goals. These goals will depend on the hospital's market competitiveness, its service delivery mix, its willingness to take on risk, and the rapidity with which managed care is growing in the community.

One or two of the three major goals of the managed care contracting effort (discussed in the following subsections) may take precedence at different times, or all may coexist simultaneously. Each goal, however, can result in a different contracting strategy.

Maintaining Current Business

The goal of maintaining current business can result in a defensive strategy, frequently due to a hospital's late entry into the managed care game. Although maintaining current business is a legitimate organizational goal, it probably is called into play *reactively*, that is, after an erosion of business was noticed. A contracting goal of maintaining current business can lead to an "I'll-do-anything-for-the-business" approach and will limit negotiating leverage.

This goal can be shortsighted because different segments of the business may be eroding. For example, a hospital's inpatient business may be healthy and growing rapidly, whereas its outpatient activity may be threatened by a managed care contract signed with a competing freestanding ambulatory surgical facility. Similarly, a hospital's laboratory, radiology, home care, or mental health business may be falling as a result of managed care contracts with competitors. This scenario can lead to a capitated agreement; the development of global fee arrangements that take into account the provision of all ancillary services; or the trade-off of lower fees for the more stable business, in return for guaranteed contracting for the eroding business.

Growing New Business

In most cases, the goal of growing new business will be chosen by an organization that has a *proactive* strategy and generally can take a tough negotiating posture. Because its core business does not seem to be under as much pressure, such an organization can hold out for more concessions during the negotiating process. This goal may also provide an organization the opportunity to be more innovative in risk taking, in that incremental business can open the door for lower average unit costs.

If the new business to be grown is in fact new business—a new product line or new service capabilities—the strategy may be even more flexible than in a situation where business is eroding. In a sense, the new product lines may be offered as "loss leaders" to establish the hospital's capabilities in these markets.

Focusing on Payer Source

As managed care expands into the Medicare, Medicaid, and worker's compensation areas, separate goals may need to be developed for each market. Aside from the issues of maintaining or growing new business, contracting for managed care business from different payer sources may have significant political implications in both the business and physician communities. This may be evident where Medicare and Medicaid are under the managed care cross-hairs and the implications of obtaining, or failing to obtain, managed care agreements can be significant for the hospital's community and its attending physicians.

For example, if a significant portion of physicians' business currently is coming from the Medicare population, and the hospital fails to embrace a Medicare managed care initiative, the physician revenue base could be threatened (as could the job of the CEO). Alternatively, an aggressive Medicare managed care initiative may not be appreciated by physicians who are prospering in the fee-for-service world. An aggressive Medicaid managed care initiative also may not be popular if physicians and board members do not fully buy into the concept and if the resulting success of the initiative changes the image of the organization in the community.

Assembling a Contracting Team

An appropriate contracting team serves both an internal and external purpose. Internally, a well-designed multidisciplinary team acts as a coordinating and educational focus for the organization and ensures that issues regarding the organization's ability to comply with the contractual agreement are addressed and brought back to the operating departments for implementation. Externally, the team assures the MCO that the appropriatere sources are available.

In some cases, this contracting team may be drawn from internal hospital staff. In other cases, members of a PHO or a joint contracting team of hospital and physician representatives may perform this function. It is the contracting team's job to understand the implications of all agreements for the operations of all the organization's units and physicians. The contracting team also must ensure that systems are in place, or will be put in place, to allow the agreement to be successful.

The size and makeup of the contracting team should differ markedly from the team that represents the provider organization in actual negotiations. This negotiating team must present the provider organization's position to the MCO and be empowered to accept terms and obligate the provider organization, and in some cases its physicians, to a final agreement. Very often, the negotiating team has only one member: a member or leader of the internal contracting team, the CEO of a PHO, or the provider organization's CEO. In some cases, a physician and administrator may comprise the team. In all instances, however, the negotiating team represents the provider organization in negotiations with representatives of the MCO. The negotiating team is supported by the internal contracting team, which provides resources to analyze the opportunities and alternatives up for negotiation. In an ideal situation, the representative areas of expertise discussed in the following subsections should be part of the contracting team and be involved in preparing for and evaluating managed care opportunities.

Finance Department

The finance department should have a good handle on the current patient mix, reimbursement rates, and profitability of various product lines. With this information, a realistic picture of the impact of any revised financial arrangement such as a discounted DRG, per diem, or global fee being offered by the MCO can be drawn. This department also should have the capability (probably with the assistance of outside actuarial advice) to assess the risk, if any, that the organization is capable of assuming and willing to assume in a potential capitated arrangement.

Physician Relations

The physician relations function may be constituted as a formal or informal organization within the hospital, such as a physicians organization (PO), independent practice association (IPA), or medical services organization (MSO), or may be represented by a PHO negotiating team. In any case, it is important to understand the implications any agreement may have for either salaried staff or attending physicians. Included here are issues related to the actual physician fee schedule being offered by the MCO, the proposed distribution of the premium dollar among the hospital and physicians, and the further distribution of the premium dollar between primary and specialty physicians.

Information Systems

As indicated earlier, one of the most important elements of any managed care arrangement is the provider organization's information systems capability. In addition to providing continuous monitoring of the financial viability of a specific managed care arrangement, an information system provides the internal mechanism to identify and modify aberrations in hospital and physician performance and build the framework for future success. Specifically, an information system can continuously profile physician performance and identify the practice patterns that lead to high-quality performance. The information system also becomes the core source for all further negotiation and strategic planning because it provides information on product line and contract profitability. Availability of an individual who understands the capabilities and limitations of the organization's information system, as well as any plans for modifying the system, is vital.

Marketing and External Relations

The marketing and external relations divisions of health care organizations historically have developed organizational relationships with local employers and community groups. Many of these relationships may change in a managed care environment, where MCOs may attempt to intercede—either through direct employer relationships or Medicare managed care contracts being offered through community groups. Nevertheless, long-standing relationships may be powerful tools in negotiating with MCOs, promoting the provider organization's involvement in managed care networks and offering support in difficult negotiations. For example, existing community programs for the Medicare population can be leveraged to support

Medicare managed care initiatives and contracts with MCOs. Similarly, a provider's long-standing relationships with employers can be used to support the provider's inclusion in a network if an MCO seeks the employers' business.

Patient Care and Nursing Services

All managed care agreements will significantly influence the manner in which patient care is provided. This is particularly the case as the need grows for improved efficiency and as issues of process and patient care reengineering emerge. Development of clinical protocols, identification of appropriate care settings, and use of alternatives such as home care are some areas that will affect patient care and nursing services. Especially profound effects will be felt where a capitated agreement is in place and all incentives are aligned to limit inpatient utilization and control inpatient costs. Such a capitated agreement will result in significant efforts to aggressively discharge patients to alternative settings and develop clinical protocols to improve patient throughput.

Quality Management and Utilization Management

As the need for enhanced operational efficiency to meet negotiated contract terms grows, so does the need to monitor both resource utilization and the impact of tighter inpatient utilization on clinical outcomes. Managed care organizations themselves are being evaluated by the NCQA using criteria such as HEDIS 2.5. It is critical, therefore, that provider organizations involved in these contract arrangements have the capability and willingness to monitor their own performance using similar criteria. Active participation of quality management and utilization management representatives in the contracting process is imperative.

Educating the Contracting Team

Of course, contracting team members should be identified for their specific knowledge of the organization and their capability to understand and implement organizational changes required as a result of managed care contracts. Team members should have analytical and team-building skills, as well as outgoing personalities, and they should be willing and able to deal with rapid change. Most important, contracting team members should be given intensive orientation to the changing world of managed care. At a minimum, this orientation should provide information about types of MCOs, types of managed care products, and changing financial risk relationships under managed care.

Turning Your Attention to the Market

Once you (and your team) have developed a comfort level with, and a clear understanding of, your organization's needs, limitations, and capabilities, you are truly ready to begin the managed care contracting process. As in any negotiation process, understanding your negotiation opponent's needs and capabilities are critical. Chapter 2 discusses how research into your potential partner's needs and capabilities should be approached by focusing on organizational characteristics, performance indicators, and network strategy.

Chapter Two

Understanding the Managed Care Organization

As managed care continues its rapid growth, so does the variety of organizations that refer to themselves as *managed care organizations* (MCOs). Although the term generally refers to health maintenance organizations (HMOs), it often is used by insurance companies and Blue Cross organizations, as well as by preferred provider organizations (PPOs) and hybrid organizations such as third-party network developers. The common denominator in all of these organizations is "the management of care," that is, the limitations placed on the insured (member) with regard to having access to any available provider—hospital or physician.

Types of Managed Care Organizations/Products

When negotiating with an MCO for its product offerings, critical considerations are the MCO's ability to control an enrolled population and guarantee that health care services will be steered in your organization's direction. Not only will this commitment vary from MCO to MCO, it will vary from product to product within a single MCO.

The following subsections describe the range of MCOs and the products they offer. In most cases, the core product offering also defines the type of MCO.

Health Maintenance Organization

An MCO must be licensed as a health maintenance organization by state regulators in order to offer this most restricted of all MCO products. A member eligible to receive HMO benefits must use *only* participating providers (hospitals, physicians, pharmacies, laboratories, and so forth) to be eligible for benefits. Use of any other providers results in no coverage. An HMO contract represents the most restrictive of all MCO products and should yield significant traffic to a

11

health care organization, unless similar HMO contracts are in place with all area providers. Providers that negotiate an agreement with an HMO, however, should expect their negotiation opponent to seek significant considerations, particularly if there are a limited number of providers under contract. As competition in the managed care market has intensified, this product has been offered in several models: primary gatekeeper, nongatekeeper, and HMO point of service.

Primary Care Gatekeeper

The member eligible to receive health benefits under this model must select a primary care physician (PCP) from a panel of participating PCPs. The PCP then is responsible for coordinating all of the member's care and must approve the services of specialist physicians, hospitals, and other providers in order for the services to be covered. In general, except for emergency services, a member receives no coverage for services not authorized by the PCP. In many cases, PCPs are reimbursed under a capitated system and may be at financial risk for specialty, diagnostic, and hospital services.

Nongatekeeper

This open-access HMO model permits members to direct themselves to specialists without prior gatekeeper approval. In most cases, PCPs in this model are reimbursed under a modified fee-for-service arrangement. Prior certification is required for utilization of certain diagnostic procedures and for elective hospitalizations, and access to providers continues to be limited to those participating with the HMO. Utilization of nonparticipating providers continues to result in noncoverage.

HMO Point of Service

In many markets, HMOs have had difficulty selling the concept of a health insurance product that limits access to providers. To ease the transition to a pure HMO product, many HMOs now offer a "point-of-service" model. In this model, a member receives full benefits if he or she uses the HMO provider network and follows the appropriate procedures (in both gatekeeper and nongatekeeper alternatives). Going outside the network of participating providers for services is permitted, however, albeit with a financial penalty of a copayment, deductible, or (in some cases) both. *Note:* Because this model affords member access to non-network providers, the probability that a contract will yield significant business correlates directly to the size of the deductible or copayment, or to the financial "pain" inflicted on the member for not using participating providers.

Preferred Provider Organizations

For the most part, preferred provider organizations act as intermediaries between insurance companies or self-insured employers and providers that deliver health care services. As a result of negotiated discounts with hospitals, physicians, and other providers, PPOs and their insurer or employer partners are able to offer an in-network and out-of-network option to those covered for health benefits. For a member to receive maximum health benefits under a PPO product, he or she must receive services from a participating provider. Covered services rendered by nonparticipating providers are covered but not to the same extent, with deductibles, coinsurance, maximums, and other similar limitations.

What is most important about agreements for PPO products is that they cannot guarantee that business will be steered to the contracting provider organization. Because in-network and out-of-network providers are easily accessible, decisions about which provider to use are totally at the member's discretion, not at the discretion of the contracting PPO entity. Most important, the majority of PPOs are not financially responsible for providing (and reimbursing for) health care benefits. This responsibility falls to the underwriting organization—either an insurance company or a self-insured employer. As a result, payment terms (for example, within 30 days) have relatively little meaning and are difficult to enforce.

Freestanding PPOs

Freestanding PPOs offer their networks of participating providers to insurance companies and self-insured employers and receive an access fee for their services as network developer and manager. Many PPOs also offer utilization management services to their clients and include significant contractual requirements that address compliance with these policies for appropriate reimbursement.

Network PPO Brokers

Network PPO brokers are organizations that may represent a number of different "payers" in their single contract. Similar to freestanding PPOs, brokers receive fees for network access. They differ from freestanding PPOs in that their contractual agreements reference multiple-payer organizations that may have different fee schedules, different reimbursement arrangements, and different utilization management programs. In most cases, these payer organizations are not even identified because they may not yet have been contracted with. Because it is impossible for providers to project potential business or limitations and constraints that may be required by each new payer, providers should not offer significant concessions.

Third-Party Administrators

Either freestanding third-party administrators (TPAs) or insurance companies offering "administrative service only" (ASO) products may fall into this category. The ASO product is offered to a self-insured employer, limiting the TPA or insurer to performing claims processing and network management functions. The TPA may have its own provider network (as may be the case with many insurers acting as TPAs) or may contract with another PPO for its network. In either case, the ultimate responsibility for claims payment falls to the self-insured employer and not to the insurer or TPA.

Performance Indicators

Before entering into negotiations with an MCO, it is important to understand as much as possible about its operations. Sources for this information include state regulatory agencies, the Securities and Exchange Commission (for publicly traded MCOs), and national directories published by organizations such as InterStudy and the Group Health Association of America. If all else fails, the MCO should be asked directly for this information. Note that in most states only HMOs are required to provide quarterly and annual financial reports, thus making it difficult to obtain comparative information for other types of MCOs.

Market Strategy and Penetration

The MCO's membership size, growth over the previous few years, managed care market share, and product line types (commercial, Medicare, Medicaid) are all important criteria in evaluating a proposed contract. This information should be made available by the MCO's marketing or provider relations staff and can be verified by checking with state regulators, employee benefits consulting firms, or national MCO directories.

The purpose here is to look at how the MCO's marketing strategy matches your organization's strategic plan and service area patient mix. An MCO targeting a commercial "yuppie" population, for example, may not have the same immediate strategic importance for an inner-city or retirement area hospital with a heavy concentration of Medicaid or Medicare patients—unless hospital leaders are making a concerted effort to attract these new populations. Similarly, a hospital that foresees its market "graying" as the service area ages may actively seek to contract with an HMO engaged in a strong Medicare marketing effort, thereby protecting and enhancing the hospital's market share.

Financial Performance

It is essential to obtain a set of the candidate MCO's financial performance indicators. These data will give a clear signal of the organization's financial viability, as well as provide utilization management and cost information. The latter in particular will be quite useful in negotiating financial terms, especially in the case of a capitated agreement. For example, if financial reports identify total hospital expenses, days of inpatient care per 1,000 members, and total number of members, a simple calculation will provide the average cost per hospital day:

Total hospital expenses = $10,000,000
Days of inpatient care per 1,000 members = 250
Total number of members = 40,000
(250 days of care ÷ 1,000 members) (40,000 members) =
  10,000 days of care
Therefore, $10,000,000 ÷ 10,000 days of care = $1,000 per day.

This is valuable information if you will be negotiating a per diem rate.

Financial ratios are useful for analyzing the financial performance of any organization, including MCOs. These ratios can help evaluate an MCO's liquidity, efficiency, asset composition, capitalization, and profitability—thus providing an instant performance "snapshot," particularly if the ratios are used to compare the organization's performance to industry benchmarks and to local and regional competitors.

Also important is the evaluation of a "moving picture" of the MCO's performance, to highlight significant favorable or unfavorable trends. Table 2-1 summarizes key financial performance indicators and industry benchmarks that can be used in the evaluation process.

As indicated earlier, sources of financial information are readily

Table 2-1. Key Financial Performance Indicators and Industry Benchmarks

Indicator	Ratio Title	Definition	Norm
Liquidity	Current ratio	Current assets divided by current liabilities	> 1.00
	Acid test	Cash and equivalent divided by current liabilities	> 0.25
	Days of premium receivables	Premium receivables divided by premium revenue per day	< 15
	Cash to claims and payables	Cash and equivalent plus premium receivables divided by total unpaid claims plus accounts payable	> 1.00
	Days of unpaid claims	Claims payable divided by medical and hospital expense per day	< 30
	Days of inpatient IBNR[a]	Inpatient IBNR divided by inpatient expense per day	< 60
	Days of physician IBNR	Physician IBNR divided by physician expense per day	< 60
	Days of referral IBNR	Referral IBNR divided by referral expense per day	< 60
	Days of other IBNR	Other medical IBNR divided by other medical expense per day	< 60
	Days of total IBNR	Total IBNR divided by related expenses per day	< 60
	IBNR as a percent of claims	Total IBNR divided by total unpaid claims	< 50%
	Claims as a percent of revenue	Total unpaid claims divided by revenue	< 15%
Efficiency	Health care delivery expense percent	Total medical and hospital expenses divided by revenue	< 85%
	Administrative expense percent	Total administrative expenses divided by revenue	< 20%
	Health care delivery expense PMPM[b]	Total medical and hospital expenses divided by member months	N/A
	Administrative expense PMPM	Total administrative expenses divided by member months	N/A
	Commercial premium revenue PMPM	Commercial premium revenue divided by member months	N/A
	Physician expense	Physician expenses divided by member months	N/A
	Hospital expense PMPM	Hospital expenses divided by member months	N/A

	Other medical expense PMPM	Other medical expenses divided by member months	N/A
	Gross margin PMPM	Premium revenue less health care expense	N/A
	Net income PMPM	Net income divided by member months	N/A
	Percent change in commercial premium PMPM	Average annual change in commercial premium PMPM	> 8%
	Percent change in health care expense PMPM	Average annual change in HCD expense PMPM[c]	< 6%
	Percent change in gross margin PMPM	Average annual change in gross margin PMPM	> 2%
	Percent change in member months	Average annual change in member month	> 1%
Asset Composition	Receivables to current assets	Premium receivables divided by current assets	< 75%
	Cash to current assets	Cash and equivalent divided by current assets	> 25%
Capitalization	Total debt ratio	Total unsubordinated debt divided by net assets	< 75%
	Debt service coverage	Net income plus depreciation and interest divided by annual principal and interest charges	> 3.00
Profitability	Net profit margin	Net income divided by revenue	> 2%
	Gross profit margin	Premium revenue less HCD expenses divided by premium revenue	> 4%
	Net worth percent change	Average annual change in net worth	> 1%

Notes: *IBNR* = incurred but not reported; *PMPM* = per member per month; *HCD* = health care delivery.
Source: Reprinted with permission from Healthcare DataBank, copyright 1993.

available. The quarterly and annual HMO reports required by state regulatory agencies identify the MCO's per-member-per-month (PMPM) costs for all health care and administrative categories and even identify some inpatient costs on a per-admission basis. In addition, regulatory filings provide detailed operating statements (including balance sheets) and show trend data from the previous year. These reports may be broken down by commercial, Medicare, and Medicaid product lines, providing valuable information that can be useful in negotiations. (A sample extract of an HMO annual report filing appears in appendix A.)

Publicly traded MCOs also file quarterly and annual financial reports with the SEC. Additional narrative information can be found in the audited financial statements and footnotes that accompany these reports. These reports also are valuable sources for information about the MCO's strategic vision and goals.

Growth Trends

A solid indicator of an MCO's market importance is its growth trend, both in terms of member enrollment and in number of clients. Of the two, the number of clients is probably the most important because it indicates the interest level in the employer community and perhaps the employee benefits consulting community—a key access point for HMO marketing efforts.

Although percentage increases may be relatively meaningless, particularly where base membership numbers are quite low, comparative data are indispensable. Enrollment information is part of all state financial reporting requirements, and key corporate client information is available in the annual report filings required by certain states. In addition, most MCO marketing departments would readily provide this information, particularly if they can point to Fortune 500 clients.

Member Satisfaction

Although most MCOs will not release member satisfaction information voluntarily, some will offer press releases when they score well in public surveys or surveys conducted by employer groups or coalitions. State information can be a valuable resource here as well, given that most states require MCOs to report member complaints and grievances. Again, this information is readily available.

A critical criterion, and a clear indicator of member dissatisfaction, is member disenrollment. Similar to employee turnover in an organization, member disenrollment can signal a problem inherent in the way an MCO operates. For example, an MCO may be doing an excellent marketing job and showing a rapid enrollment rate, but it may be doing a poor job operationally and losing members at the same (or faster) rate. Particularly in cases of rapid growth, the MCO may not have the infrastructure to provide adequate services to its customers (who also include physicians and hospitals). Therefore, because an MCO's growth may be short-lived, providers interested in contracting opportunities should be armed with enrollment (and disenrollment) data to better evaluate the MCO's long-term potential.

Contracting Requirements

If you've seen one MCO, you've seen one MCO. Each MCO has a personality and corporate culture of its own. Whether that culture is one of collaboration or institutional arrogance may be sensed during initial contact with the provider relations representative. Furthermore, the prevailing culture can become standardized with the MCO's approach to negotiations—for example, developing an "off-the-shelf" contract offered at the opening round.

With some MCOs, even contract terminology is indicative of the culture. For example, substituting legalese (*whereas, heretofore*) and impersonal labels (*contractor, contractee*) with more humanistic terms such as *we* and *you* suggests a unique and refreshing approach and may be a preliminary indicator of a collaborative approach. The following paragraphs, which describe responsibilities of the hospital and the MCO, is one such example:

> You will make those health care services available which are described in the applicable coverage documents on the same basis as you do for your other patients. You will make these services available for our covered persons, as defined in the exhibits.
>
> You will give us and state and federal agencies access at reasonable times upon request to your books, records and papers concerning the health care services you provide to our covered persons, the charge of the services, the payments received by you from our covered persons (or from others on their behalf), and your audited financial statements.

Chapter 3 details the significance of each contract term used in a final negotiation.

During the initial assessment of an MCO agreement, it is important to look for the level of cooperation or authoritarianism implied in the initial contract and for those approaches or procedures required by the MCO that may not be politically or philosophically acceptable in your organization. This general assessment can be useful as an additional criterion in setting initial negotiating priorities.

Following are general issues to keep in mind during this compatibility analysis:

- *Authorization requirements:* How restrictive is the MCO in terms of its requirements for inpatient admission, emergency care, diagnostic testing, and referrals?
- *Records/data requirements:* How demanding is the MCO with respect to requiring records, reports, and access to your files?
- *UM/QA management:* How invasive is the MCO's medical management program with respect to on-site reviews, physician profiling, credentialing requirements, and access to committee minutes?
- *Billing/reimbursement:* How cumbersome is the billing process? How restrictive are the fee schedules? What guarantees are there for claims turnaround? How will capitations be developed?
- *Accessibility:* How will interactions with the MCO be handled? Who is the liaison, and what involvement will staff and physicians have in the development of guidelines and operational policies?
- *Patient interaction/education:* How will the MCO deal with hospital–patient interactions regarding the MCO? This can include everything from requiring patient education programs, to limiting staff responsibility, to criticizing MCO operations.

Provider Network Strategy

It is critical to understand an MCO's provider network strategy if your contracting goal is to develop a long-term strategic partnership. Very often, an MCO's contracting strategy correlates directly to the product line it plans to offer. Many MCOs offer multiple products and have multiple provider networks in what can be described as a concentric circle arrangement.

The product with the most restrictive provider access—usually a low-priced HMO—will have a number of low-priced (or deeply discounted) hospitals at the circle's core. Beyond this inner core may be a second tier of "preferred" hospitals that, again, either have lower prices or offer reasonable discounts. The outer tier often contains the balance of all hospitals in a region and is probably offered as part of a point-of-service, or "freedom-of-choice," option.

The goal of all contract negotiations is to reach the inner core of providers in order to ensure patient activity for all of the MCO's products. You must understand not only the characteristics of "inner-core" providers, but the MCO's current approach and future plans for products and providers alike.

For those providers that have not made the cut for the inner core, it is important to understand the criteria on which this decision was based so as to identify which performance characteristics may need improvement to reach that level, if desired. Because the potential for significant patient activity relates directly to a provider's position within the MCO network, so too should the concessions your organization is willing to offer in contract negotiations.

Rolling Up Your Sleeves

Now that the difficult soul searching and intensive homework is completed, you are ready to begin the negotiation process. Chapter 3 describes key operational (nonfinancial) contract elements you should be mindful of when undertaking a negotiation effort. The chapter also provides detailed analysis of each contract component and recommended terms.

Chapter Three

Negotiating the Contract: Key Operational Considerations

It is important to begin this chapter by strongly advising every organization or individual contemplating negotiation of a managed care contract to obtain the services of qualified legal counsel. Although contract terms can be negotiated from a performance and operational point of view, many areas require expert legal advice. By the same token, it is important to realize that a thorough legal analysis of a contract may not necessarily take into account many operational and political issues that can strongly influence the completion or rejection of a managed care agreement.

The following contract negotiation analysis is presented from a layperson's perspective and does not factor in the number of legal nuances that may apply to your specific situation. It does, however, examine key elements that appear, or should appear, in every managed care agreement. Also provided are detailed explanations of the various contract components and descriptions of an array of negotiating positions for each component, ranging along a spectrum from best, to good, to worst.

Contract Elements: Evaluating the Terms

Contract terms generally cover six areas. They include parties to the agreement and products covered, reimbursement terms and conditions, operational obligations, renewal and termination provisions, post-termination obligations, and amendments.

Parties to the Agreement and Products Covered

Given the growth of managed care and the preponderance of entities now calling themselves managed care organizations (MCOs), it is imperative to quickly determine what type of MCO you may be dealing with. As described earlier in this book, the major contracting organizations that may call themselves MCOs include health maintenance organizations (HMOs); national or regional insurance companies, including Blue Cross plans; and third-party network developers and administrators that offer preferred provider organization (PPO) products. Each one may offer multiple product lines that have very different implications for an organization contemplating a contractual agreement. These product lines may include the following:

- A pure HMO product with network access limited to contracted providers only
- A point-of-service (POS) product with access to nonparticipating providers, albeit with a financial penalty of deductible, coinsurance, or maximum fee schedule
- PPO product with provisions similar to a POS product but no distinct "captured" population of covered lives
- An administrative services only (ASO) product for self-insured employers, with financial responsibility at the employer level and no financial risk to the insurer
- Hybrid models of any or all of the preceding products

You should understand how each product operates, what restrictions it imposes, how patients are steered to contracting parties, and (most important) how your organization can identify which product covers a given patient.

Health Maintenance Organizations

Health maintenance organizations are unique among all MCOs in that they are explicitly regulated by individual states, usually by the state's commissioner of insurance. In fact, the National Association of Insurance Commissioners (NAIC) has developed regulatory guidelines that, for the most part, are similar from state to state and are used to monitor HMO financial and operational performance. In some states, regulatory responsibility is shared with the state health department, which examines and monitors issues such as access to care, patient satisfaction, and quality of care.

Health maintenance organizations may offer multiple products including a pure HMO, a POS product, and hybrids. In addition, HMOs may offer products marketed to the Medicare and Medicaid populations under capitation agreements with federal or state governments. In some states (such as New York), HMO-type organizations (referred to in New York as *prepaid health services programs* [PHSPs]) have been licensed to provide services only to the Medicaid population. Although such organizations are licensed and regulated in a manner similar to standard HMOs, they may contract only for Medicaid enrollees.

What is distinctive about contracting with HMOs is the amount of performance and operations information available. As discussed earlier, your team needs a solid understanding of the candidate MCO to develop an effective negotiations strategy. As regulated organizations, MCOs must file quarterly and annual financial statements with their state insurance commissioners. These reports may be obtained directly under a state's freedom of information act at a cost per copied page, or they may be obtained from third parties that collate and summarize data for all HMOs licensed in a state.

Such reports can assist with the following initiatives:

- Evaluating the HMO's financial viability
- Identifying the HMO's medical expenses, administrative expenses, and profits
- Identifying the HMO's premium competitiveness
- Identifying the HMO's growth trends

National or Regional Insurance Companies

Nationally recognized insurance organizations such as Aetna, Cigna, Prudential, and local and regional Blue Cross plans may have state-regulated HMOs among the array of products they offer. In addition, they may have insurance-based PPO and POS products and, most important, a significant number of ASO agreements with their clients. With these products, self-insured employers are offered contracted networks of providers and claims-processing services. A considerable amount of this business will come from larger national employers seeking local networks for their local employees. What is most significant about these arrangements is that self-insured products are the financial responsibility of the employer, not the insurer or MCO. Thus, any contractual agreement that offers a provider network to a self-insured employer is only as financially viable as the employer that contracts for the services. It is imperative, then, to know which employers are currently under contract and to monitor the contractual arrangements between the MCO and its clients. Doing so ensures that the MCO is not contracting with financially unstable organizations and passing on the financial risk of health care expense collection to its network participants.

Third-Party Network Developers and Administrators

Third-party network developers and administrators are a hybrid category of MCOs, and in most states they have new formal legal status. In essence, network developers act as brokers, representing clients that may be insurance companies or employers negotiating with providers on a direct contract basis. For all intents and purposes, the products offered by third-party developers are PPOs. These MCOs normally have a contract with their clients to develop a preferred network of providers. They also may be obligated to pay claims and/or institute some type of utilization review program. Some network developers have the capability to pay claims, but others contract with third-party administrators (TPAs). *Third-party administrators* are claims payment organizations that may develop their own provider networks or contract with network developers to jointly package a product for an employer. In many instances, these MCOs have no obligations whatsoever, leaving the provider to fend for itself in the event problems arise with a client insurance company or employer.

The clearest indicator that an MCO is in fact a third-party network developer or administrator is appearance of the term *payer* in the contract. As in the case of an insurer acting under an ASO agreement, it is important to determine who the payers are so that it can be comfortably established that these organizations are financially solvent and reliable. In cases where these contractual arrangements are put in place to represent more than one insurer or employer, it is important to build a mechanism into the contract that allows for termination of services with one insurer or employer should problems arise, but without jeopardizing the overall contractual arrangement with other insurers and employers.

It is also important that you and your organization's team understand the relationship between a third-party developer and its clients. If this type of MCO has no ongoing obligations for utilization management (UM), a contracting provider is at the mercy of multiple UM programs that may be in place in each of the MCO's client insurance companies or employers—a situation that can present an operational nightmare. On the other hand, if the MCO has UM responsibilities, only one set of guidelines and procedures will require adherence.

Reimbursement Terms and Conditions

The reimbursement section of the contract being analyzed deals with issues related to claims submission and payment under a fee-for-service contractual arrangement. For organizations entering into capitation arrangements, claims submission issues may not be relevant although, similar to claims, requirements maybe in place for submission of "encounter" information. Claims payment obligations for capitation arrangements should focus on when the capitated payment is due and the type of supporting information (describing the number and type of "covered lives") to be provided by the MCO in order to reconcile the capitation payment.

Claims Submission

Issues related to claims submission generally include time frame, format, and supporting documentation. These are described briefly in the following subsections.

Time Frame

Claims submission time frame has significant financial implications for a provider. This section of the contract normally requires that bills be submitted within a set time frame to be eligible for payment. Timely submission of bills allows the MCO to accurately predict its incurred but not reported (IBNR) expenses, thereby enabling it to assess more accurately its current financial performance. Managed care organizations may propose that claims not received within a reasonable time be denied. Time frame is negotiable.

When this language is included in a contract, your organization should agree on clear terms that reflect the facility's current billing capabilities and ability to determine whether a patient is a member of the MCO in question. If possible, have this section eliminated altogether.

Worst Terms:	Short time frame for submission (30 days). No payment for late submissions.
Good Terms:	90+ days for submission and/or no penalty for late submission.
Best Terms:	Provider will make "best effort" to submit claims within 120 days, or no reference in contract at all. No penalty for late submission.

Claim Format

Many contracts start the claims payment turnaround clock from the point at which "a completed claim in an acceptable format" is received. Under these terms, no financial obligation is incurred until this point. Thus, it is important to clearly identify what billing format is acceptable and standardize it in the contract.

Worst Terms:	Format "acceptable" to health plan, with no form specified.
Good Terms:	Standard UBF or HCFA 1500 forms.
Best Terms:	Electronic and/or manual submission of claims at provider's discretion.

Supporting Documentation

Many MCO contracts request documentation to support claims submitted. This is particularly true when a claim for emergency services is submitted, where copies of emergency department (ED) summaries and/or records are requested as supporting material. In addition to being an operations problem (for example, retrieving copies of records for certain payers), it can be quite costly both in terms of personnel and copy costs.

Worst Terms:	Documentation required for all claims. No reimbursement for copies of records.
Good Terms:	Verification information provided on an as-needed or sample basis. No individual retroactive denials of claims. Fees for record copies.
Best Terms:	No reference made. No specific requirements. A request for documentation for retrospective review is not punishable by claim denial. Copy costs are reimbursed.

Claims Payment

Claims payment issues generally include turnaround time, billing restrictions, eligibility notification, benefit limitations, payment obligations, retrospective denials, compensation, remittance statements, and prior authorization.

Turnaround Time

When evaluating an MCO agreement, it is as important to look for items missing as it is to examine terms included. Most MCO agreements will not address the MCO's obligations to make timely payments, so it is imperative to include language that clearly specifies what is expected from the MCO. In contracts with network developers and PPOs, ascertain that the obligations the MCO is committing to are also being committed to by the payer organizations with which it contracts. This is critical because the MCO in these cases has no financial obligations.

> *Worst Terms:* No reference, therefore no commitment.
> *Good Terms:*   Within 30–90 days of bill receipt.
> *Best Terms:*   Within 15–30 days of bill receipt.

Patient Billing Restrictions

Under most states' HMO regulations, patients are "held harmless" in the event an HMO fails to make payments to providers. This hold-harmless provision does not apply to deductibles and coinsurance payments that an HMO member is obligated to pay.

Some MCOs and HMOs offering non-HMO products are seeking similar hold-harmless provisions and may be vague as to how deductibles and coinsurance issues are addressed, seeming to hold patients harmless for those payments as well. Where network developer and PPO organizations are involved, it may be unclear who has what obligation to pay and when, and whether the patient may be billed—even for deductibles and coinsurance.

> *Worst Terms:* Language that prohibits patient billing in the event neither MCO nor payer pays, even for non-HMO patients.
> *Good Terms:*   Limits hold-harmless provisions to HMO patients.
> *Best Terms:*   Limits hold-harmless provisions to HMO patients. Ensures ability to bill patients for non-HMO product lines when plan does not pay. Clearly allows for billing of deductibles and coinsurance.

Member Eligibility Notification

When a member enrolls in an MCO—more important, when a member terminates membership—has significant financial implications to the provider. Therefore, the contractual agreement must provide a clearly delineated mechanism for identifying current members, as well as the products under which those members are covered. The contract also should provide for regular updates of enrollment information and clearly specify how and when a member becomes personally liable for health care charges.

In capitation relationships, an explicit reconciliation process should be included. This will require regular scheduled reports that identify member additions and deletions, with specific cutoff dates (for example, the 15th of every month). These monthly reports should be reconciled with the required monthly documentation that should accompany the MCO's capitation payment.

> *Worst Terms:* No commitment to membership updates.
>   Ability to retrospectively deny payments
>   for nonmembers, even where MCO did not
>   provide information.
> *Good Terms:*   Monthly membership listing updates.
> *Best Terms:*   Membership card. On-line electronic
>   verification of membership. No retrospec-
>   tive denials if MCO makes an error.

Coordination of Benefit Limitations

Although the coordination of benefit (COB) provisions of most managed care contracts are difficult to read, the concept is simple. The
MCO is attempting to limit the amount of money it spends on a
member's claim in situations where the member has other insurance coverage. In doing so, it attempts to limit its financial exposure
(or that of its clients).

When the MCO acts as a secondary payer (another insurer has
the primary obligation), an attempt is usually made to limit the
provider's ability to collect beyond what would have been paid if the
MCO was the primary payer. This can be significant if the MCO has
negotiated a discount while the primary payer has not. When the
MCO acts as a primary payer, contract language may limit what the
provider can collect from a secondary payer. Contract language should
stipulate what the provider can do with regard to secondary payers,
regardless of who the secondary payer is.

> *Worst Terms:* Limits collection from secondary payers to
>   maximum of what would be paid by MCO.
> *Good Terms:*   When MCO is secondary, additional billing
>   is limited to maximum of bill after primary
>   reimbursement, subject to MCO maximum
>   coverage.
> *Best Terms:*   When MCO is secondary, additional billing
>   is allowed up to maximum coverage,
>   regardless of primary reimbursement. No
>   limitations on secondary billing when
>   MCO is primary.

Obligations to Pay

The obligations to pay clause is most important when dealing with
network developers and PPOs. Although these organizations have
no legal obligation to make payments if they are representing third-
party payers (insurers, employers, unions, and so forth), a mechanism for arbitrating problems should exist, and the network devel-

oper should be obligated to play some type of intermediary role in the event one of its clients has not made payments either at the appropriate level or in a timely fashion.

Also crucial is the status of the entire contract in the event that a single third-party payer fails to meet its obligations. Provisions in either the contract or the termination section should permit dropping a single payer without jeopardizing the entire agreement and the relationships with other payers.

Worst Terms:	No role for network developer if payer fails to pay. Patient cannot be billed.
Good Terms:	Network developer plays role as arbitrator. Patient can be billed.
Best Terms:	Network developer assumes liability for payment and/or patient can be billed directly. Payer can be terminated without jeopardizing agreement.

Retrospective Denials

In entering an agreement, the managed care organization is seeking certain controls over utilization of the provider's services. The provider should be seeking a long-term relationship that benefits both parties. Retrospective denials are punitive measures, and they should not be acceptable in contractual relationships. The basic principle underlying the contractual relationship—both parties agree to provide certain services and perform certain obligations on a timely and effective basis—should be clearly laid out in advance. If either party is unhappy with the other's performance, the contract should be terminated.

Worst Terms:	Punitive retrospective denials for "inappropriate" utilization and/or lack of documentation. No ability to appeal.
Good Terms:	No retrospective denials if prior authorization is received. Ability to appeal.
Best Terms:	No retrospective denials. Process in place to identify and correct problems.

Compensation

Although this area may overlap with topics covered earlier, compensation may be a separate component in a managed care contract and therefore is discussed as a discrete clause here. Whether intentional or unintentional, compensation language in managed care agreements tends to be vague with regard to coinsurance and where bills have not been paid by the MCO. This is often the case when different products are covered by a single contract.

Under most state licensing regulations, members must be "held harmless" in the event that a licensed HMO fails to pay its bills. This provision serves to protect covered individuals should the HMO become insolvent. Bear in mind (and in the contract) that in no way does the provision free a member from obligation to pay for any deductibles or copayments. As indicated earlier, it is important to try to limit hold-harmless provisions to licensed HMO products only.

Worst Terms:	Allows "hold harmless" to encompass deductible, coinsurance, and non-HMO products.
Good Terms:	Clear language allowing billing for any patient deductibles and coinsurance.
Best Terms:	"Hold harmless" is limited to HMO products. Clear language allowing billing of patient for deductibles and coinsurance.

Remittance Statements

The absence of a provision for remittance statements is significant. (A *remittance statement* is a summary report that accompanies MCO payments and describes reimbursements and rejections of claims covered by the payment.) From an operations perspective, the managed care contract should require that the provider receive regular reports describing payments by product line, claims denials by coded reason, and any claims that may be pending subject to review. This will allow the provider's accounts receivable staff to monitor payment accuracy and validate the rate and/or discount being applied.

In addition, if claims are being "pended" for review purposes, it is important to know why in order to develop internal procedures to avoid similar problems in the future. Monitoring pended claims has a secondary effect: Managed care organizations with cash flow problems may attempt to slow payments by pending more claims for review. Monitoring these trends can provide an early warning signal of potential problems with the MCO and allow your organization to trigger contract compliance and/or termination clauses.

Worst Terms:	No commitment in contract to provide remittance statements.
Good Terms:	Remittance statements provided on an infrequent and/or less-than-detailed basis.
Best Terms:	Remittance statements provided monthly

on the status of all submitted claims for all product lines covered by the agreement.

Prior Authorization

The MCO's rationale for prior authorization is an important negotiation issue. Prior authorization is a critical component in the coordination-of-care process, whether it is done by the MCO, the primary care physician (PCP), or both. It is also an important control aspect for those providers considering capitation arrangements.

The verification process ensures that an admission or referral is medically necessary for the entity absorbing the financial risk. It also triggers any utilization management activity that attempts to limit length of stay, particularly where a per-diem inpatient agreement is in place. Finally, the authorization process identifies an admission for the MCO's financial projections of IBNR expenses well before a claim is submitted.

A contractual relationship with a high-quality MCO should not call for "punishment" if the provider fails to obtain prior authorization for what otherwise would be an appropriate and medically necessary admission. Sometimes, however, contracting with an MCO that has these stringent requirements may be necessary in the short term to meet strategic objectives. Generally speaking, endorsing punishment of a partner could signal an MCO approach that would not bode well for a long-term relationship.

On the other hand, keep in mind that authorization requirements are legitimate for the above-described purposes. A provider unwilling or unable to comply with these legitimate business requirements is not an acceptable partner to an MCO.

> *Worst Terms:* Onerous requirements that will punish and otherwise not tolerate or accommodate a minor administrative infraction, even if the service provided is deemed medically necessary and appropriate.
>
> *Good Terms:* Reasonable language that clearly defines prior authorization requirements and establishes a reasonable level of error tolerance prior to financial or other penalties.
>
> *Best Terms:* Reasonable language that clearly defines prior authorization requirements but does not penalize provider for medically necessary and appropriate services.

Operational Obligations

This section deals with the important but frequently neglected hospital obligations to meet an MCO's reporting, auditing, and other requirements. These requirements can significantly strain your staff, particularly where contracts are in place with several MCOs. Some of these operational obligations are briefly described in the following subsections.

Medical and Other Records

A number of records-related issues frequently appear in MCO contracts, including record retention, MCO access to records, and confidentiality of records. Not always limited to medical records, MCO requests may include copies of minutes of various committees to assure the MCO that certain activities (credentialing, utilization management, quality management, and so forth) are taking place per the agreement.

Record Retention

Efforts should be made to limit the MCO's record retention requirements to those mandated by state or federal regulatory agencies or, where MCO requests are more stringent, to the hospital's own record retention policies.

> *Worst Terms:*   Unlimited retention of records.
> *Good Terms:*   Specified time period agreed to in advance.
> *Best Terms:*   Limited to state regulatory requirements.

Access to Records

Many MCOs request unlimited access to records solely at their convenience. Such an obligation would wreak operational havoc in a hospital and add significant staff costs, particularly if multiple MCO contracts are in place, with any number of individuals traipsing through the hospital's record rooms. Access to records should be restricted and controlled under terms of the contract agreement.

Although a request for *copies* of records seems less imposing, copies are much more problematic and costly from an operational perspective. Managed care organizations may try to reduce their costs and increase their surveillance by requesting that copies of records be attached to certain bills (such as those for emergency services). This activity should be severely restricted in any agreement.

Worst Terms: Unlimited access. No fee imposed for copies.

Good Terms: Limited access with advance notice and during normal business hours.

Best Terms: No access to records on-site. Copies of records only, with a reasonable fee imposed per copy.

Confidentiality

Medical records should be made available only with appropriate patient authorization. Making the record request process too simple can result in requests for records that really may be unnecessary but "nice to have," transferring the administrative burden (and inherent cost) to your organization. Records of quality assurance and utilization management committees, as well as physician credentialing activities, should not be provided; if they must be provided to verify compliance, it should be stipulated that identifiers will be removed.

Worst Terms: No reference made to patient authorization. Unlimited additional information requested.

Good Terms: Generic patient authorization built into MCO membership application, and copy sent with each request for medical record. No additional information made available to MCO beyond items required by state or federal regulatory agencies.

Best Terms: Patient authorization presented for each medical record request if possible. No additional information made available to MCO beyond items required by state or federal regulatory agencies.

QA/UM Program Compliance

Agreeing to abide by an MCO's quality assurance (QA) and utilization management programs without seeing these plans in advance is tantamount to driving blindfolded. Because each of these plans has numerous requirements and obligations, it is important to review them in advance and have them formally added to the agreement as addenda. That way, your organization knows beforehand what is being agreed to. Any changes to the QA or UM plan, then, should be treated like any other contract modification or addendum.

As in the preceding discussion of reports, information, and committee minutes, requests for QA and UM minutes often appear in the QA and UM plans. Confidentiality issues must be kept in mind here. Minutes should not be provided or, in the worst case, identities should be protected.

Utilization management plans may call for retrospective denials of claims if UM procedures are not complied with, an approach that should not be acceptable. A hospital–MCO agreement should call for relationship building and "partnering" around contract compliance. Punishment for noncompliance does not foster that type of relationship. The hospital should be given notice of noncompliance as it occurs. If the MCO continues to be unhappy with the hospital's compliance with its UM or QA requirements, it has the right to terminate the agreement.

Finally, the MCO may not be meeting procedural obligations, such as preadmission certification and notification of emergency admission, in a timely fashion. The agreement should clearly delineate these obligations and ensure that the burdens of compliance within a specific time frame (for example, notification within 24 hours) do not fall on the hospital if the MCO is at fault.

Worst Terms:	General "agree to comply" language in the agreement.
Good Terms:	UM/QA policies and procedures are attached to the agreement as formal addenda. Modifications may be made only with prior notification.
Best Terms:	UM/QA policies and procedures are attached to the agreement as formal addenda. Modifications may be made only by amending the agreement.

Licensing and Accreditation Reports

Many MCOs seek to utilize the hospital's Joint Commission on Accreditation of Healthcare Organizations (JCAHO) accreditation reports as part of the selection criteria for participation in their network or on an ongoing basis to assist the MCO's quality assurance efforts. These reports are highly confidential and should not be released. Information released should be limited to copies.

Similarly, MCOs may request copies of notifications of regulatory or licensing violations. In fact, they are asking you to utilize your own resources to provide negative reports on your performance. Although your reaction to these requests might seem obvious, you do have an obligation to be licensed and accredited and should be responsible for documenting your status.

Worst Terms:	Requirement to provide copies of all JCAHO findings and to notify MCO of any action against the hospital that could jeopardize its licensure.
Good Terms:	Requirement to provide copies of licensing and accreditation certificates. Requirement to notify MCO of any formal action taken by regulators.
Best Terms:	Requirement to provide copies of licensing and accreditation certificates only.

Miscellaneous Notification and Compliance Requirements

Careful review of each MCO request in a proposed agreement will identify a number of items that are unnecessary, readily conceded by the MCO, and easily negotiated away. These items can range from notification of a malpractice claim filed, to the forwarding of monthly financial statements. Even agreements that obligate the hospital to "not undermine the confidence of members in the HMO" are not unheard of. The administrative burden of providing these items is apparent. In negotiations, the simplest way to eliminate many such requests is to ask for similar information from the MCO (monthly financials, rate filings, and so forth). Nevertheless, reasonable information (for example, annual financial statements, an updated medical staff list) can and should be provided.

Worst Terms:	Very detailed and specific requests for significant amounts of information, for example, individual malpractice claims and regular reports. Responsibility for controlling situations largely beyond the organization's influence (such as incidents of employee criticism of the MCO in front of patients).
Good Terms:	Reasonable compliance requirements, including summary and outcome information (for example, malpractice claim settlements).
Best Terms:	Limited, reasonable compliance requirements.

Equity of Obligations

Often overlooked during negotiations is the fact that *two* parties are involved, each having certain obligations to the other. Generally, however, the "hospital obligations" section of a proposed agreement is more exhaustive than the "MCO obligations" section—if one exists at all. It is reasonable to request, therefore, that any section of the agreement that calls for a hospital obligation be met with an equal MCO obligation.

Parity of obligation applies to reporting requirements, amendments and terminations, and any other area that can be identified clearly. This approach in a negotiation session helps establish a collaborative atmosphere and is a valuable strategy for eliminating some of the unnecessary obligations referred to in preceding sections.

> *Worst Terms:* No MCO obligations. One-sided approach.
> *Good Terms:*   Reasonable reporting requirements and comparable obligations.
> *Best Terms:*   Line-by-line matching of reporting and notification procedures.

Contract Renewal and Termination Provisions

This section addresses MCO provisions that deal with agreement extension, termination, post-termination obligations, and modification. It is interesting to note that weeks, if not months, are spent on negotiating the fine details of MCO agreements, only to find that the agreement has a unilateral 90-day termination clause. In fact, what has been negotiated is a 90-day contract. The following subsections expand a bit on the importance of these terms.

Renewal

In general, contracts should be limited to one year, with provisions made for renewing them well before termination date. Where automatic renewal is proposed, provisions should be made for adequate time to assess and amend financial and reimbursement issues at least annually.

In special instances, multiyear contracts should be considered if they provide extraordinary opportunities. Note, however, that the managed care environment continues to be volatile, so that long-term commitments may carry significant risk, particularly where costs can change dramatically in a short time. Furthermore, in an environment where MCO acquisitions and consolidations are commonplace, the MCO originally contracted with may be gobbled up by another organization.

Worst Terms:	Automatic renewal unless terminated. No reference to modification of rates/reimbursement.
Good Terms:	Automatic renewal unless terminated. Renegotiation of rates 90–180 days prior to renewal date.
Best Terms:	Year-to-year renewal. Renegotiation of rates 90–180 days prior to renewal date.

Termination

Termination provisions should be carefully spelled out and distinguish between termination "for cause" and termination "without cause." As discussed in the subsection on equity of obligations, termination provisions should be the same for both parties. Your team should seek clarification for "with-cause"termination provisions and negotiate for an arbitration methodology for resolving problems that otherwise could lead to termination.

A contract having a "without-cause" termination notification period of 90 days is in effect a 90-day contract and should be dealt with accordingly with regard to other terms. This short-term "bailout" holds important implications for a hospital if an MCO begins to face financial problems. In a highly competitive market, MCOs may be forced to price their products at rates they cannot sustain and may be under severe financial pressure for up to 12 months while their rates remain in effect. The first signal of a cash-starved organization is a slowdown in claims payment. If financial performance does not improve, your hospital does not want to be left holding the financial bag (as many did when MCOs went bankrupt). The 90-day termination clause circumvents that risk.

Worst Terms:	One way, 30 days without cause by MCO.
Good Terms:	180 days without cause by either party.
Best Terms:	90 days without cause by either party.

Post-Termination Obligations

Very simply, all hospital obligations should terminate upon termination of the agreement, except for continuity-of-care concerns. Managed care organizations may ask to continue their financial arrangements while they find a replacement or until they can move their patients. In the best case, all discounted and/or special reimbursement arrangements should terminate as well, even if patients remain hospitalized.

Your organization may want to temper its position in this area, depending on who terminated the agreement. If the hospital terminates the agreement, some provision may exist for continuity of reimbursement arrangements for those hospitalized members. If the MCO terminates the agreement, a tougher stance may be appropriate.

> *Worst Terms:* Care provided for 180 days after termination, at contracted rates.
> *Good Terms:* Care provided at contracted rates through discharge date.
> *Best Terms:* Care provided at contracted rates through termination date.

Amendments

During agreement negotiations, much time and effort is spent carefully reviewing each item, but significant changes are frequently made through the amendment process. Amendments may be clear-cut changes in core contract performance or reimbursement obligations, or they may be changes in peripheral requirements in operating manuals that could significantly affect the hospital's ability (or willingness) to continue its contractual relationship. An example of this situation is an amendment that changes the content of reports to include the identities of physicians against whom malpractice claims have been filed. Such a change could be made in the utilization review manual instead of the formal agreement and be instituted without receiving appropriate scrutiny.

Any significant change to an operating procedure and/or manual should be deemed an amendment to the basic agreement. Appropriate notification should be provided prior to an amendment, and either a positive action (signature on the amendment) or an explicit ability to reject an amendment—without jeopardizing the agreement—should be provided for.

> *Worst Terms:* Amendment process is by letter from MCO. Amendment takes effect in 30 days.
> *Good Terms:* Amendment process is by letter from MCO. Amendment takes effect in 60 days unless other party objects.

Best Terms: 30-day advance notice of amendment by
either party. Formal notification and
approval required for any amendment.

Drop-Dead Issues

Every negotiator and organization has an individual tolerance limit
that, if exceeded, means walking away from a deal. Some MCO contracting issues clearly require a hard line and a tough and unrelent-
ing stance. Usually these issues involve limitations on the way your
organization conducts future business, add unacceptable legal liability, or involve policies or procedures that threaten the organization's
continued viability (or the CEO's job). Some of these issues are sum-
marized below:

- *Most-favored nation clause:* This clause mandates that any
  terms you negotiate with another MCO must automatically
  be offered to the one with which your organization is negotiating, regardless of all other considerations. This approach
  ties the hospital's hands in future negotiations with all other
  parties. In some cases, there may be no other choice if the
  MCO's failure to execute or terminate your agreement could
  result in a financial or operational disaster—all the more reason to carefully plan your overall negotiations strategy.
- *Exclusivity:* Some MCOs may request an exclusive arrangement, requiring that you do not contract with any of their
  competitors. This is another approach that ties the hospital's
  hands and limits its future strategic and negotiating flexibil-
  ity. Exclusivity is particularly important given the volatile
  environment of MCO mergers and acquisitions. Tying your
  organization's future to the financial and operational success
  of an other organization is not an appropriate strategy.
- *One-way indemnification:* Although this issue calls for a
  more in-depth discussion with your legal counsel, suffice it
  to say that an approach that holds your organization liable
  for an MCO's inappropriate behavior (even malpractice)
  should not be tolerated.
- *Patient confidentiality:* An MCO unwilling to accept the
  stringent patient confidentiality requirements that you and
  your legal counsel desire is probably not an organization to
  develop a long-term relationship with; the MCO may not
  convey to its staff your strong commitment to confidential-

ity. Breaches of patient confidentiality are more probable if large numbers of your records circulate among hundreds of MCO employees. Any breach could result in serious and irreparable damage to your organization's reputation.

Getting to the Bottom Line

The issues surrounding MCO contracting terms are multidimensional and complex. Any negotiating process involves determining what criteria are important to you and making concessions in less-important areas. To illustrate the big picture of an MCO agreement, two contracts are presented in appendix B for comparison purposes. The first contract is with the "World's Oldest Renowned Simply Terrific Health Plan, Inc." (the "WORST Health Plan") and shows how some of the least provider-friendly terms would appear in an agreement. The second agreement, with the "Great Old Original Doctors Health Plan, Inc." (the "GOOD Health Plan"), illustrates how some of the terms from the WORST agreement have been modified to be more provider friendly. Modifications appear in *italic type* for easy identification.

Regardless of an agreement's contractual terms, success, failure, and future financial viability will rest on the financial terms your team negotiates. Chapter 4 details key financial terms in an MCO agreement.

Chapter Four

Negotiating the Contract: Key Financial Considerations

Although operational considerations are important in managed care contracting, financial considerations are paramount. Financial performance is critical to an MCO's competitive position and even more essential to for-profit, publicly traded MCOs that must respond to Wall Street investor demands and expectations. From a hospital's perspective, the financial parameters of an MCO agreement are critical to the hospital's financial viability. The financial section of the proposed contract deserves your closest attention.

It is important to define and describe the multitude of financial arrangements that currently prevail in MCO agreements. Each option carries a certain element of risk, both for the MCO and the contracting hospital; each tends to evolve from less risk to more risk in individual geographic markets. Therefore, familiarity with the spectrum of financial risk arrangements is essential because the more risk-laden agreements no doubt will arrive in your markets—if they have not already done so.

When thinking about the risk attached to MCO arrangements, do not overlook the counterbalancing *reward* element. This concept, which may seem relatively simple, is often forgotten by hospitals that fail to take reward opportunities into account, concerning themselves only with the bottom-line risk. Ironically, such "risk-averse" organizations frequently offer discounted fee-for-service arrangements to MCOs and learn too late that they cannot sustain the discounts. They end up offering a risk arrangement with no reward opportunity.

Your organization's willingness to accept risk correlates directly to some of the tough organizational self-assessment questions raised in chapter 1. Nevertheless, it is important to keep in mind that by not accepting risk you might severely limit your reward potential.

Low-Risk Reimbursement Methodologies

Three reimbursement methodologies carry lower levels of risk: fee for service and discounted fee for service; per-diem arrangements; and case payments (DRGs and global fees).

Fee for Service and Discounted Fee for Service

Fee for service and discounted fee for service are the preferred methods of reimbursement among most hospitals first entering into managed care contracting agreements. These arrangements carry the least financial risk exposure and, for the most part, have the least impact on hospital operations. Usually, a hospital offers the MCO a discount off its charges for both inpatient and outpatient activity on the assumption that the MCO will refer more patients to the hospital to take advantage of the discount.

The hospital must continue to show a profit on each discounted service, and an increase in volume must in fact lead to an increase in surpluses. Although it may be difficult to quantify the projected overall financial impact of a managed care agreement, losses on individual services cannot be made up for in volume.

Per-Diem Arrangements

Per-diem arrangements have become the most prevalent reimbursement arrangement offered for inpatient hospitalization because they can take advantage of the MCO's aggressive utilization management efforts to control hospitalizations. As discussed earlier, an important performance criterion for an MCO is its inpatient days per 1,000 members. Aggressive, successful MCOs have lowered commercial inpatient days per 1,000 members to less than 200 in some areas of the country. Not too long ago the accepted standard was 500–600 days per 1,000 members for a similar population.

A *per diem* is a flat fee for each day of a patient's hospital stay. Per diems offer a hospital minimal risk (and reward) because a "profit" can be earned if the per-diem costs are lower than the rate negotiated. Similarly, a loss can be incurred for each day that the per diem is lower than the hospital's true costs.

A per-diem financial arrangement combined with an aggressive utilization management program can have a significant positive financial impact on MCO performance. Similarly, this combination can have an equally significant *negative* impact on a hospital's financial performance—unless the rates are negotiated skillfully and the volume of business from the MCO truly increases.

Many MCOs will negotiate per-diem arrangements using the hospital's average length of stay as a basis. Thus, hospitals with longer lengths of stay will receive lower per-diem rates and stand to be most vulnerable when lengths of stay are reduced by the MCO's utilization management efforts. Therefore, your organization must understand the methodology used by the candidate MCO to calculate per diems so that appropriate rates can be negotiated.

Per-diem arrangements can be negotiated for different service lines (obstetrical, medical, surgical, and any other special services) if supporting data are available to identify the cost differentials. In a similar way, MCOs may be open to negotiating what are known as "L-shape" per diems, where a higher rate is paid for the initial days of a stay to take into account the higher costs generated by the extensive care provided to the patient, and a lower flat rate is offered for subsequent days wherein services are relatively limited.

The simplest example of this kind of arrangement is a normal obstetrical delivery. Many MCOs will offer a flat per-diem arrangement and work hard to discharge the patient in two to three days. Because most of the hospital's overhead and operational expense occurs on the day of delivery, it is important to load the first day's per diem with all of these expenses. Beyond the delivery day, the hospital is really providing "hotel" services, and the per diem could be lowered to cover those expenses.

A hospital's financial exposure in this arrangement is limited if the MCO discharges the patient quickly because the bulk of the expenses, incurred during the first day, have been covered by the loaded per diem. Obviously, such an arrangement is more beneficial to the hospital because it limits financial exposure.

In situations where an MCO is new to a region and does not have a large database, your hospital may have a stronger negotiation position because of its information base. In these situations, the MCO may be using state or regional data to develop its per-diem rate. In any case, having a strong data-based negotiating position can be effective in both initial and renewal negotiations.

Case Payments

Under case payment arrangements, the hospital is paid a single fee for all services provided to a patient during one hospital stay or one clinical care episode (that is, a surgical procedure). This distinction is significant in financial negotiations because a patient may be readmitted for complications during an otherwise single episode of care.

In most cases, the MCO will use DRG categories because these are familiar and easily understood. Although case payments fix the payments for all hospital services, global fees include the physician fee in the packaged price. Often these payments are made for highly specialized tertiary procedures (such as open-heart surgery and transplants) and offer significant opportunities for exclusive arrangements.

Case payments contain some of the same minimal incentives and risk-sharing opportunities found in per diems but go a step further in that they offer an incentive for the provider to voluntarily reduce length of stay. This additional incentive, of course, is balanced by an additional risk because a longer length of stay, regardless of the reason, will not receive additional reimbursement.

High-Risk Reimbursement Methodologies

Although the actuarial and accounting issues surrounding a high-risk reimbursement methodology like capitation payments are relatively complex, the concept is simple. Capitation is a prepayment for health care services based on a flat rate per person (per capita) paid on a regular basis, usually monthly. When payment is capitated by an MCO, a hospital is paid a specific amount per member per month (PMPM) to provide a particular set of services to its assigned members.

InterStudy, a national managed care information resource and consulting firm, compiled 1995 information into a report entitled *InterStudy Competitive Edge* (Industry Report 5.1; Waltham, MA: Decision Resources, Inc., 1995, p. 70). The study found that 25 percent of HMOs use capitation as a hospital reimbursement method, an increase from 18 percent in 1994. InterStudy's findings also indicated, however, that three out of five HMOs that capitate hospitals reimburse less than 20 percent of all hospital services with this method. Thus, although capitation is becoming more prevalent, its impact continues to be limited to a small portion of most hospitals' overall business, even within the limited scope of MCO agreements. Capitation agreements are becoming the dominant method of reimbursement, however, in regions with higher levels of managed care penetration and where significant reduction in hospital days of care has already taken place.

In addition to purely capitated agreements, other reimbursement arrangements offer risk- (and reward-) sharing opportunities. The following discussion of capitated and other risk-based methodologies, although not an in-depth financial and actuarial treatment, is meant to show that the complexities and risks inherent in these agreements are significant and should not be undertaken without serious financial analysis and expert advice from consultants or actuaries.

Capitation Agreements

Under a capitated agreement the hospital receives a fixed payment each month for each member, but most members assigned to that hospital will not require services in any given month. If claims for services are less than the capitated payment, the hospital shows a short-term "profit"; if claims exceed the capitated payment, the hospital shows a short-term "loss."

Because capitated payments are based on projected expenses relative to probability factors and expectations related to utilization and the demographic mix of the enrolled population, profit and loss must be evaluated on a longer-term basis to allow for the statistical probabilities to take their course. Financial reports that show high profit or high loss in the short term will not have much meaning until an agreement has been in place for 6 to 12 months. This slower-than-normal evaluation time frame presents a financial control problem and increases the risk potential.

Because the impact of an inappropriate capitation cannot be assessed for a number of months, potential losses may be high. In addition, any intervention required to rectify the problem, such as renegotiating the capitation rate or decreasing operating costs, will be significantly delayed, thereby increasing the financial loss. So it is imperative that these agreements be carefully monitored on a timely basis, that short-term losses be monitored for continued trends and rapid intervention, and that short-term profits not generate a false sense of security.

Capitated payments may be limited to hospital services or may include all health care services provided to a population, including physician care, ambulatory care, and diagnostic services. Under such agreements, the incentives and profit-sharing arrangements of all providers receiving reimbursement must be aligned to ensure that any savings generated—by more improved utilization, shorter lengths of stay, or more aggressive use of home care that limits hospital days—are shared by all who can control them. Making this happen is easier said than done, both from an operational and political perspective, and is a topic beyond the scope of this book.

Withholds

Many physicians involved in managed care are familiar with the withhold method of risk sharing. In this arrangement, an agreed-on percentage of either a capitated or fee-for-service payment is placed in a separate account as incentive to control utilization. Reimbursement of the withhold is conditioned on the attainment of certain financial or utilization performance conditions.

Withhold arrangements constitute risk sharing, as opposed to profit sharing, because the best the hospital can do is retrieve 100 percent of its negotiated financial terms. The withhold, however, does provide a way to limit risk by capping the total financial exposure to the amount set aside in the withhold pool.

Clearly, then, negotiating a withhold provision in an MCO agreement should be approached in the exact same manner as a discounted fee arrangement in evaluating its potential financial impact. The levels of risk your institution is willing to accept under these types of arrangements should be tied to the percentage being withheld, the conditions for distributing the withhold, and the hospital's ability to influence the performance necessary to achieve those conditions.

Risk Pools

Managed care organizations often establish risk pools as an alternate method of sharing risk with providers. Under a risk pool arrangement, the MCO allocates a specific amount per member per month for specialty services, emergency services, and inpatient care. These funds are deposited into risk pool accounts and are drawn on if utilization does not meet expected targets.

Risk pools normally are used in global fee or capitation-type arrangements to give physicians a financial stake in the costs resulting from their practice decisions. Appropriately designed risk pools also help hospitals modify the practice behavior of physicians who generate inpatient expenses the MCO must pay from the hospital's funds.

If a hospital's funds are not in a risk pool, it is important to determine whether the physicians' funds are. Physician risk pool arrangements can affect hospital financial performance significantly, because physicians will be highly motivated to reduce hospitalizations and emergency services utilization.

Controlling or Limiting Risk

Despite the significant differences among the various risk arrangements, one thing remains clear: In any risk-based arrangement, the MCO has effectively transferred to the hospital and its affiliated providers a portion of the financial risk. As licensed and heavily regulated insurers, MCOs have significant experience and resources to evaluate the actuarial risk they face, whereas most hospitals do not. Therefore you should become familiar with the many strategies (discussed in the following subsections) for controlling financial risk and build these safeguards into contractual negotiations as well as implementation activities.

Evaluating the Rate

In evaluating a proposed capitation-based risk agreement, it is important to determine whether the capitation rate offered is reasonable and adequate. A significant source of risk in a capitated agreement is the statistical fluctuation inherent in predicting hypothetical membership levels and service utilization. Statistical fluctuation will decrease as the number of members covered by the agreement increases.

A capitated agreement is built around multiple assumptions concerning average medical costs, utilization, age and gender distribution of the enrolled membership population, and so forth. Because they are assumptions, uncertainties in these parameters are inevitable and are exacerbated by the following conditions:

- Historical data are limited.
- Changes are made in the benefit plans.
- Services covered under the capitation are unclear.
- Incorrect assumptions are drawn about trends (including the demographic mix of members and out-of-network utilization).
- The effects of new utilization management and provider incentives are unknown.

Your negotiation team must carefully scrutinize the assumptions an MCO makes in developing capitations or risk pools. At a minimum, capitated agreements should be calculated based on the exact age and gender distribution of the hospital's covered population. Because the final mix of patients will remain uncertain, it is important to develop a multitiered capitation rate so that a specific rate will be applied to each demographic group. This way, the hospital is assured of receiving a higher rate, for example, for females in their 20s expected to demonstrate high utilization levels and a lower rate for males in the same age group with lower utilization levels.

Obviously, the most difficult part of evaluating the adequacy of a proposed capitation rate is to accurately project utilization and cost of services for the enrolled MCO population. There are two ways to markedly limit uncertainty in these projections.

The first involves doing your own extensive analysis using publicly available information or information provided by the MCO. As mentioned earlier, much information is available from state regulatory reports, rate filings, and national managed care organizations such as the Group Health Association of America. Financial statements will show the actual expenses paid by the MCO for inpatient, physician, and other health care, in terms of both actual per member per month and percentage of premiums (see appendix A, pp. 62–63). The MCO's annual report or rate filing usually will identify the actual and/or expected age and gender distribution of the covered population, as well as the projected health care expenses for each category. An example of this segment of the report appears in appendix A, pp. 66–67. Such information is critical for determining an accurate rate.

The second way to project utilization and cost is the easier and more costly alternative of hiring an outside actuarial firm. Advantages to using external actuarial resources include their access to large databases of utilization rates and costs; their ability to use forecasting models; their expertise in actuarial science; and their experience with MCOs, which may use them to develop premium rates.

Carve-Outs

One commonly used method for limiting or controlling risk is the introduction of carve-outs. As implied, this strategy "carves out" of the capitated or risk agreement certain high-cost services or procedures that may not easily be controlled by the hospital or that, because of their low probability of occurring, could present serious financial problems. Examples of these high-cost, low-probability categories include transplants and open-heart surgical procedures. An actuarially determined value for these services is deducted from the financial agreement, and their cost is borne by the MCO.

Another way in which a carve-out can be implemented is by identifying a high-risk category of patients and eliminating them from the risk arrangement. For example, patients who have AIDS, hemophilia, or substance abuse problems may be excluded because of the high volume (and cost) of services they utilize. As with the procedure categories, an actuarially determined value for such patient populations is deducted from the financial agreement, and the cost for these services is borne by the MCO or subcontracted to an organization that specializes in providing such services.

Generally speaking, the carve-out approach is acceptable to the MCO because it understands what actuaries refer to as the "risk of small numbers," and because of its own ability to "spread" the financial risk over a larger member base. This risk refers to the potentially devastating financial impact of a high-cost case when there is only a small base of premium-paying members. One high-cost case can instantly wipe out months of capitated payments (or, in the MCO's case, premiums).

Stop-Loss Insurance

By definition, risk-based agreements are risky, and it is neither possible (nor desirable) to eliminate all financial risk. As in most situations where financial risk is a factor, *insurance* is the practical remedy, specifically stop-loss insurance, or reinsurance.

Here again, the name implies the definition. Stop-loss insurance limits hospital exposure to unforeseen and unpredictable high-cost cases and "stops the loss" at a set amount. Stop-loss insurance can be obtained on an individual patient basis (total claims per patient of $50,000, for example) or on an aggregate basis (that is, taking into account the total expenses for the entire covered population).

Stop-loss insurance limits financial exposure when legitimate care exceeds a specific threshold. It does so by providing reimbursement at a predetermined level (80 percent or 100 percent) once expenses exceed the threshold. By eliminating the possibility of claims reaching catastrophic levels, it fixes the upper level of costs, thereby fixing the maximum loss and risk. Because a premium is charged for the insurance on a per-member per-month basis, stop-loss insurance also lowers the potential reward.

Improving Operational Performance

Most capitated or risk-sharing negotiations use performance data of the hospital or its regional competitors as a baseline for determining the financial arrangement. By definition, much risk is uncontrollable and depends on best-guess actuarial assumptions of patient mix and expected utilization. Other financial risk—specifically, the financial risk related to your organization's clinical operations performance—can be controlled.

Recall that a capitated rate is based on expected utilization patterns and costs of delivering health care services, expectations that derive from historical performance information. Clearly, then, by outperforming the utilization assumptions underlying the capitation rate, the hospital and its physicians not only can limit their risk significantly, but also enhance the reward probability.

Implementation and Performance Monitoring

Once a contract has been signed and its terms are being implemented, an internal control and monitoring system should be put in place to assess what impact the contract is having on the organization. This monitoring system should be overseen by members of the managed care contracting team, who should be accountable for reporting the effect of managed care agreements on their respective departments. At minimum, a monitoring system should look for the following indicators:

- *Financial performance:* First and foremost, the financial impact of the MCO agreement should be monitored carefully. Parameters include timeliness of claims or capitation payments; overall projected versus actual revenue; and, within limitations of the time frame required in capitated agreements, profitability of the agreement to your organization.
- *Market share impact:* Issues here include whether the business provided by the MCO represents new patients or the same patients at different rates; whether the patient mix (commercial, Medicare, Medicaid) has changed; and whether significant changes have occurred in the hospital's service area—with patients coming from outlying or new geographic areas.
- *Operational impact:* Issues to be monitored here include the administrative burden imposed on hospital staff by this new agreement, including record requests, problems at admission, utilization management programs, problems with early discharges, and overall relations with MCO staff.
- *Physician impact:* It is critical to monitor how affiliated physicians feel about the MCO agreement, both from a financial and "hassle factor" perspective. The best of all MCO agreements will fail dismally if physicians are unhappy with their arrangement.

A Continuous Improvement Process

The managed care contracting process is not unlike the continuous quality improvement process familiar to most organizations. Not only will new MCOs surface in most markets, but hospitals will aspire to new performance and risk levels as they become more familiar with the managed care field.

A well-conceived process for negotiating contracts and monitoring contract performance will be essential to your organization's success. This process should include the following components:

- Ongoing assessment of your organization's strengths and weaknesses
- Ongoing assessment of the MCOs in your marketplace
- A carefully thought-out set of operational and financial criteria for contract negotiation and renegotiation
- A monitoring and feedback system for ongoing performance evaluation of the agreements

With such a process in place, your organization can increase its chances for thriving in a managed care environment. Good luck!

Sample HMO Annual Report Filing (Extract)

HMO Annual Report

Name of HMO HMO One Health Plan, Inc.	For the Period Ending December 31, 1994

Report #1—Part A: Balance Sheet (Assets)

	Current Period	Previous Year
Current Assets		
1. Cash[a]	$44,337,221	$61,929,139
2. Short-term investments	0	0
3. Premiums receivable—net	3,537,511	3,854,618
4. Interest receivable	260,168	29,252
5. Other receivables—net	481,972	333,389
6. Prepaid expenses	0	0
7. *Total current assets* (Items 1 to 7)	$48,616,872	$66,146,398
Other Assets		
8. Restricted assets	$ 310,000	$ 300,000
9. Restricted funds	568,299	862,926
10. Loan escrow	0	0
11. Long-term investments	12,361,033	0
12. Intangible assets and goodwill—net	0	0
13. Leasehold improvements—net	0	0
14. Rental security	48,021	48,021
15. *Total other assets* (Items 9 to 15)	$13,287,353	$ 1,210,947
Property and Equipment		
16. Land	$ 0	$ 0
17. Building and improvements	0	0
18. Construction in progress	0	0
19. Furniture and equipment	0	0
20. *Total property and equipment—net* (Items 17 to 21)	$ 0	$ 0
21. *Total assets* (Items 8, 16, and 22)	$61,904,225	$67,357,345

[a]Cash and cash equivalents include participation in a corporate cash management program.

HMO Annual Report

Name of HMO	For the Period Ending
HMO One Health Plan, Inc.	December 31, 1994

Report #1—Part B: Balance Sheet (Liabilities and Net Worth)

	Current Period			Previous Year
	1 Covered	2 Uncovered	3 Total	4
Current Liabilities				
1. Accounts payable	$ 160,154	$ 0	$ 160,154	$ 146,067
2. Claims payable (reported)	9,779,700	0	9,779,700	9,923,929
3. Accrued inpatient claims				
(not reported)	7,217,609	0	7,217,609	11,270,122
4. Accrued physician claims				
(not reported)	2,056,606	0	2,056,606	790,548
5. Accrued referral claims				
(not reported)	0	0	0	0
6. Accrued other medical	3,900,917	0	3,900,917	6,171,543
7. Accrued medical incentive pool	362,940	0	362,940	82,394
8. Unearned premiums	492,550	0	492,550	817,776
9. Loans and notes payable—				
current	162,000	0	162,000	149,000
10. Other current liabilities	16,502,024	0	16,502,024	19,631,086
11. Total current liabilities	$40,634,500	$ 0	$40,634,500	$48,982,465
(Items 1 to 10)				
Other Liabilities				
12. Loans and notes	$ 1,044,000	$ 0	$ 1,044,000	$ 1,206,000
13. Statutory liability	0	0	0	0
14. Total other (escheat liability)	215,192	0	215,192	242,800
15. *Total other liabilities*	$ 1,259,192	$ 0	$ 1,259,192	$ 1,448,800
(Items 12 to 15)				
Net Worth				
16. Donated capital	XXX	XXX	$ 0	$ 3,891,796
17. Capital	XXX	XXX	1,000	1,100
18. Paid in surplus	XXX	XXX	4,880,140	4,880,040
19. Reserves and restricted funds	XXX	XXX	0	0
20. Unassigned surplus	XXX	XXX	15,129,393	8,153,144
21. *Total net worth* (Items 16 to 20)	XXX	XXX	$20,010,533	$16,926,080
22. *Total liabilities and net worth*			$61,904,225	$67,357,345
(Items 11, 15, and 21)				

HMO Annual Report

Name of HMO	For the Period Ending
HMO One Health Plan, Inc.	December 31, 1994

Report #2: Statement of Revenues and Expenses

	Budgeted Amount	Current Period	Variance Amount
Revenues			
1. Premium	$177,467,000	$133,765,706	$(43,701,294)
2. Fee for service	0	0	0
3. Copayments	0	0	0
4. Title XVIII—Medicare	0	0	0
5. Title XIX—Medicaid	0	0	0
6. Interest	1,363,000	2,726,302	1,363,302
7. C.O.B. and subrogation	2,702,000	1,577,540	(1,124,460)
8. Reinsurance recoveries	0	587,216	587,216
9. Other revenue	13,100,000	17,980,255	4,880,255
10. *Total revenue* (Items 1 to 9)	$194,632,000	$156,637,019	$(37,994,981)
Expenses (Medical and Hospital)			
11. Physician services	$ 56,290,000	$ 36,854,457	$ 19,435,543
12. Other professional services	0	0	0
13. Outside referrals	0	0	0
14. Emergency services, out-of-area, other	31,231,000	12,009,932	19,221,068
15. Occupancy, depreciation, and amortization	0	0	0
16. Inpatient	42,429,000	31,820,066	10,608,934
17. Reinsurance expenses	0	494,538	(494,538)
18. Other medical	13,873,000	12,803,514	1,069,486
19. Incentive pool adjustment	0	0	0
20. *Total Medical and Hospital* (Items 11 to 19)	$143,823,000	$ 93,982,507	$ 49,840,493
Administration			
21. Compensation	$ 18,958,710	$ 16,110,554	$ 2,848,156
22. Interest expense	306,000	602,961	(296,961)
23. Occupancy, depreciation, and amortization	3,820,676	3,257,468	563,208
24. Marketing	4,597,080	4,051,254	545,826
25 Other	2,516,606	7,905,481	(5,388,875)
26. *Total Administration* (Items 21 to 25)	$ 30,199,072	$ 31,927,718	$ (1,728,646)
27. *Total Expenses* (Items 20 and 26)	$174,022,072	$125,910,225	$ 48,111,847
28. *Income (Loss)*	20,609,928	30,726,794	10,116,866
29. Extraordinary item	0	0	0
30. Provision for taxes	7,214,000	10,777,236	(3,563,236)
31. *Net Income (Loss)*	$ 13,395,928	$ 19,949,558	$ 6,553,630

HMO Annual Report

Name of HMO HMO One Health Plan, Inc.	For the Period Ending December 31, 1994

Schedule S-7 Hospitalization Expenses

Inpatient Services: Contracting Hospital (List)	Cost of Services Provided	Average Cost per Day	Average Cost per Admission
1. Medical Center A	$ 7,731	$ 773	$ 7,731
2. Hospital B	48,570	1,150	2,136
3. Community Hospital C	195,548	1,003	3,810
4. Hospital D	8,867	2,956	4,433
5. Medical Center E	134,315	1,281	3,460
6. Memorial Hospital F	287,204	1,080	2,849
7. Medical Center G	304,261	963	6,170
8. Hospital H	160,989	933	2,736
9. Medical Center I	32,484	1,015	2,499
10. Medical Center J	189,409	1,023	4,603
11. Community Hospital K	810	810	810
12. General Hospital L	243,995	1,345	4,452
13. Medical Center M	300,291	1,295	2,613
14. Community Hospital N	427,882	1,134	2,480
15. Medical Center O	147,723	1,698	5,276
16. Hospital P	75,295	1,237	2,351
17. Medical Center Q	125,356	1,435	3,486
18. Medical Center R	33,292	972	2,041
19. Medical Center S	1,582,043	1,037	3,481
20. Medical Center T	74,419	1,618	3,721
21. Medical Center U	137,097	837	2,160
22. Medical Center V	36,283	1,134	2,791
23. Medical Center W	65,884	1,345	3,876
24. Memorial Hospital X	129,118	1,927	6,796
25. Medical Center Y	151,467	1,040	2,989
26. Memorial Hospital Z	4,919,972	1,406	5,419
27. Hospital AA	108,377	1,088	2,448
28. Medical Center BB	525,513	1,146	4,285
29. Medical Center CC	641,856	1,070	3,426
30. Memorial Hospital DD	842,227	1,129	2,785
31. Medical Center EE	143,754	2,178	15,973
Subtotal	$12,082,031		

HMO Annual Report

Name of HMO	For the Period Ending
HMO One Health Plan, Inc.	December 31, 1994

R-1 Ambulatory Encounters by Type and Membership Status
Summary Table

Type of Ambulatory Encounter	Number of Encounters by Members[a]	
	Total (a)	Average Number per Member per Year (b)
1. Medical care—total		
A. Physicians (excluding psych.)	244,181	3.51
B. Nurses		
2. Mental health services (includes psych.)		
3. Dental health services		
4. Other direct services—total		
A. Alcohol abuse referral and treatment		
B. Drug abuse referral and treatment		
C. Home health (skilled nursing)	2	0.00
D. Health education		
E. Medical social services		
F. Laboratory	814	0.01
G. X ray		
H. Emergency		
In-area	9,686	0.14
Out-of-area		
I. Other (please specify) misc. services	21,752	0.31
5. *Total ambulatory encounters*	276,435	3.97

[a]Count each encounter only once and assign to the appropriate category based on the principal services rendered and the reason for the encounter. Include only encounters for covered services.

HMO Annual Report

Name of HMO
HMO One Health Plan, Inc.

For the Period Ending
December 31, 1994

R-2 Utilization of Inpatient Services by Total Membership
Summary Table

Type of Inpatient Services[b]	Total Admissions		Total Days Hospitalized		Hospital Days	
	From Contracting Facility[a] (a)	From Noncontracting Facility[a] (b)	In Contracting Facility (c)	In Noncontracting Facility (d)	Total (e)	Per 1,000 Members (f)
1. Hospital total						
A. Medical/surgical	2,927	626	13,686	3,735	17,421	250
B. Obstetrical (maternity)	903	194	1,908	518	2,426	35
C. Newborns in hospital[c]	873	189	2,480	702	3,182	46
D. Mental health (psychiatry)	42	9	7	165	874	12
E. All other						
2. Skilled nursing facility total						
3. Intermediate care facility total						
4. *Total inpatient days*	4,745	1,018	18,783	5,120	23,903	343

[a] A *contracting facility* is a facility that has a contract with the HMO to provide services for a specified fee or capitation. These facilities should be listed in question Q-1.
[b] If more than one health condition is treated during the hospital stay, the plan should determine the one condition considered to be primary with respect to the hospitalization and report the case accordingly.
[c] Newborn days should be reported separately from obstetrical days. Count each newborn day as a full day even if it is billed as a part of the mother's stay.
Note. Days hospitalized should be total days before coordination of benefits.

HMO Annual
Schedule K—Recapitulation—Part 1
HMO One Health Plan, Inc.

A Regular Membership Excluding Medicare and Medicaid	B Current Year	C Previous Year
1. Enrollment		
1.1 Member months per year	1,202,450.00	1,001,858.00
1.2 Contract months per year	468,806.00	387,599.00
1.3 Average family size	3.83	3.81
1.4 Average contract size	2.28	2.51
1.5 Contract mix	2:5	2:5
1.6 Individual contract months	191,446.00	149,198.00
1.7 Husband & wife contract months	32,275.00	19,777.00
1.8 Family contract months	245,085.00	218,624.00
2. Premiums		
2.1 Basic premium charged:		
2.2 Individual	$125.61	$120.05
2.3 Family	$317.17	$303.14
2.4 Ratio (individual/family)	1:2.50	1:2.50
2.5 Coinsurance charged (per visit to H.C.)		
3. Income		
3.1 Basic premium (pm/pm)	$100.22	$95.33
3.2 Riders premium (pm/pm)	$0.57	$0.49
3.3 UDC		
3.4 Prescription drug	$10.70	$9.38
3.5 Optical		
3.6 Dental		
3.7 Other	$0.00	$0.00
3.8 Total rider capitation (pm/pm)		
3.9 Investment income (pm/pm)	$0.71	$0.73
3.10 Fee for service (pm/pm)		
4. Other revenue		
Loans:		
4.1 Federal		
4.2 Other		
Health service (per 1,000 enrollees)		
included Medicare and Medicaid		
4.3 Number of FTE physicians		
4.4 Number of FTE other medical personnel		
4.5 Inpatient days	$39,868.00	$30,182.00
4.6 Ambulatory encounters	$405,901.00	$377,174.00
5. Expenses		
5.1 Medical service (pm/pm)	$52.23	$49.94
5.2 Medical occupancy & overhead (pm/pm)		
5.3 Hospital—inpatient (pm/pm)	$24.82	$28.00
5.4 Outside medical (pm/pm)	$1.42	$1.70
5.5 Outpatient (pm/pm)	$6.11	$4.59
5.6 Emergency room (pm/pm)	$5.13	$3.86
5.7 Referral (pm/pm)		
5.8 Laboratory (pm/pm)		
5.9 X ray (pm/pm)		

6. Administrative expenses
   6.1 Marketing cost (pm/pm) $0.82 $0.94
   6.2 Administrative cost (pm/pm) $7.96 $6.72
   6.3 Occupancy and overhead (pm/pm) $0.64 $0.50
   6.4 Debt service (pm/pm) $0.01 $0.00

7. Ratios
   7.1 Ratio of current assets to current liabilities   0.972   0.873
   7.2 Average length of stay—regular   4.503   4.105
   7.3 Average length of stay—Medicare
   7.4 Average length of stay—Medicaid   3.681   4.139

HMO Annual Report
Schedule K—Recapitulation—Part 2
HMO One Health Plan, Inc.

A Regular Membership Including Medicare and Medicaid	B Current Year Amount ($)	%	C Previous Year Amount ($)	%
Revenues				
1. Basic premium by contract	133,384,037	96.68	104,904,252	97.67
2. (1)	0	0.00	0	0.00
3. (2)	0	0.00		0.00
4. (3)	0	0.00	0	0.00
5. (4) Medicare premium	0	0.00	0	0.00
6. Rider income	686,418	0.50	495,378	0.46
7. Medicare	0	0.00	0	0.00
8. Medicaid	3,040,347	2.20	1,277,285	1.19
9. Fee for service	0	0.00	0	0.00
10. Investment income	848,229	0.61	731,596	0.68
11. All other revenue	0	0.00	0	0.00
12. *Total revenue*[a]	137,959,031	100.00	107,408,511	100.00
Expenses				
13. Physician services[b]	64,034,529	46.42	50,600,669	47.11
14. Inpatient	28,965,692	21.00	28,468,711	26.51
15. All other medical	29,319,307	21.25	17,506,546	16.30
16. *Total hospital and medical*	122,319,528	88.66	96,575,926	89.91
17. Administration	11,841,131	8.58	8,279,052	7.71
18. *Total expenses*	134,160,659	97.25	104,854,977	97.62
19. Net income (loss)	3,798,372	2.75	2,553,534	2.38
20. Other revenue	0		0	
21. Net income (loss)	3,798,372	2.75	2,553,534	2.38
22. Projected break-even enrollment				

[a] Total revenue = 100% of all other items related to total revenue.
[b] Includes other professional services and outside referrals.

HMO Annual Report
Report #4—Part B: Projected Revenues and Expenses
HMO One Health Plan, Inc.
(Excluding Medicare and Medicaid for Each Line of Business)

Member Months	1st Quarter 326,285		2nd Quarter 329,267		3rd Quarter 334,809		4th Quarter 337,151		5 Total 1,327,512	
	$	PMPM($)	$	PMPM($)	$	PMPM($)	$	PMPM($)	$	PMPM($)
Revenues										
1.1 Premium (basic) community rated	33,850,506	103.75	34,143,347	103.70	34,692,734	103.62	34,921,390	103.58	137,607,977	103.66
1.2 Premium (basic) class rated	0	0.00	0	0.00	0	0.00	0	0.00	0	0.00
1.3 Premium (drugs)	3,517,430	10.78	3,546,959	10.77	3,609,088	10.78	3,632,569	10.77	14,306,046	10.78
1.4 Premium (other riders)	153,914	0.47	157,629	0.48	161,857	0.48	165,546	0.49	638,946	0.48
2. Fee for service	0	0.00	0	0.00	0	0.00	0	0.00	0	0.00
3. Title XVIII—Medicare (HCFA)	XXX	XXX	XXX	XXX	XXX	XXX	XXX	XXX	XXX	XXX
4. Title XIX—Medicaid (state & federal)	XXX	XXX	XXX	XXX	XXX	XXX	XXX	XXX	XXX	XXX
5. Investment	179,457	0.55	181,097	0.55	184,145	0.55	185,433	0.55	730,132	0.55
6. Aggregate write-ins for other revenues	0	0.00	0	0.00	0	0.00	0	0.00	0	0.00
7. Total revenue (Items 1 to 6)	37,701,307	115.55	38,029,032	115.50	38,647,824	115.43	38,904,938	115.39	153,283,101	115.47
Expenses										
Medical and Hospital										
8. Physician services	18,045,705	55.31	18,202,183	55.28	18,494,234	55.24	18,615,510	55.21	73,357,632	55.26
9. Other professional services	0	0.00	0	0.00	0	0.00	0	0.00	0	0.00
10. Outside referrals	0	0.00	0	0.00	0	0.00	0	0.00	0	0.00
11. Emergency room, out-of-area, other	4,483,291	13.74	4,524,813	13.74	4,601,056	13.74	4,632,782	13.74	18,241,942	13.74
12. Occupancy, depreciation, and amortization	0	0.00	0	0.00	0	0.00	0	0.00	0	0.00
13. Inpatient	8,303,937	25.45	8,376,414	25.44	8,513,554	25.43	8,569,942	25.42	33,763,847	25.43
14. Incentive pool and withhold adjustment	0	0.00	0	0.00	0	0.00	0	0.00	0	0.00

		Amount	%	Amount	%	Amount	%	Amount	%	Amount	%
15.	Aggregate write-ins for other medical and hospital expenses	147,716	0.45	148,977	0.45	151,342	0.45	152,325	0.45	600,360	0.45
15.1	Drug expense	3,517,430	10.78	3,546,959	10.77	3,609,088	10.78	3,632,569	10.77	14,306,046	10.78
15.2	Rider expense	153,914	0.47	157,629	0.48	161,857	0.48	165,546	0.49	638,946	0.48
16.	Subtotal (Items 8 to 15)	34,651,993	106.20	34,956,975	106.17	35,531,131	106.12	35,768,674	106.09	140,908,773	106.15
17.	Reinsurance expenses net of recoveries	97,512	0.30	98,407	0.30	100,062	0.30	100,749	0.30	396,730	0.30
18.	Copayments	0	0.00	0	0.00	0	0.00	0	0.00	0	0.00
19.	C.O.B. and subrogation	808,805	2.48	818,437	2.49	835,041	2.49	841,807	2.50	3,304,090	2.49
20.	Subtotal (Items 18 and 19)	808,805	2.48	818,437	2.49	835,041	2.49	841,807	2.50	3,304,090	2.49
21.1	Total medical and hospital (Items 16 and 17 less 20)	33,940,700	104.02	34,236,945	103.98	34,796,152	103.93	35,027,616	103.89	138,001,413	103.95
21.2	Revenue less medical and hospital (Item 7 less 21.1)	3,760,607	11.53	3,792,087	11.52	3,851,672	11.50	3,877,322	11.50	15,281,688	11.51
	Administration										
22.	Compensation	2,110,035	6.47	2,128,189	6.46	2,162,602	6.46	2,177,487	6.46	8,578,313	6.46
23.	Interest expense	2,587	0.01	2,609	0.01	2,651	0.01	2,670	0.01	10,517	0.01
24.	Occupancy, depreciation, and amortization	210,518	0.65	212,330	0.64	215,763	0.64	217,248	0.64	855,859	0.64
25.	Marketing	227,981	0.70	229,942	0.70	233,660	0.70	235,269	0.70	926,852	0.70
26.	Aggregate write-ins for other administrative expenses	682,649	2.09	688,522	2.09	699,655	2.09	704,472	2.09	2,775,298	2.09
27.	Total administration (Items 22 to 26)	3,233,770	9.91	3,261,592	9.91	3,314,331	9.90	3,337,146	9.90	13,146,839	9.90
28.	Total expense (Items 21.1 and 27)	37,174,470	113.93	37,498,537	113.88	38,110,483	113.83	38,364,762	113.79	151,148,252	113.86
29.	Income (loss) (Item 7 less 28)	526,837	1.61	530,495	1.61	537,341	1.60	540,176	1.60	2,134,849	1.61
30.	Extraordinary items (explain)	0	0.00	0	0.00	0	0.00	0	0.00	0	0.00
31.	Provision for federal income taxes	0	0.00	0	0.00	0	0.00	0	0.00	0	0.00
32.	Net income (loss) (Item 29 less Items 30 and 31)	526,837	1.61	530,495	1.61	537,341	1.60	540,176	1.60	2,134,849	1.61

Note: Unfavorable variances should be indicated by parentheses around the amount. Significant unfavorable variances of $0.50 or more should be explained in a narrative attachment.

HMO Annual Report
HMO One Health Plan, Inc.

Schedule 1—Enrollment Data (Participants)
(For Each Line of Business or Area)
All Regions

A	B	C	D	E	F
	Prior Year End	1st Quarter	2nd Quarter	3rd Quarter	Current Year End
1. Employer groups	0	0	0	0	0
1a. Class rated	0	0	0	0	0
1b. Community rated	147,726	163,495	167,212	172,003	175,136
2. Medicare	0	0	0	0	0
3. Medicaid	1,879	2,628	3,605	4,053	4,511
4. *Total*	149,605	166,123	170,817	176,056	179,647

Schedule 2—Membership Total HMO by Age and Gender

A Age	B Total	C Male	D Female
1. Under 1	2,912	1,461	1,451
2. 1–4	13,329	6,83	6,494
3. 5–14	32,159	16,591	15,568
4. 15–19	13,478	6,948	6,530
5. 20–24	12,141	5,067	7,074
6. 25–44	67,335	29,808	37,527
7. 45–64	34,321	16,007	18,314
8. 65 & over	3,972	1,959	2,013
9. Unknown	0	0	0
10. *Total*	179,647	84,676	94,971

Note: The total of schedule 1, column F, should agree with the total of schedule 2, column B.

Schedule 3—Total HMO Medical Cost Analyzed by Age and Gender

	A Age	B Total ($)	C Male ($)	D Female ($)	E Total PMPM($)	F Male PMPM($)	G Female PMPM($)
1.	Under 1	4,628,541	2,593,086	2,035,455	2.26	1.27	0.99
2.	1–4	7,577,032	4,284,525	3,292,507	3.70	2.09	1.61
3.	5–14	12,787,47	6,827,132	5,960,340	6.25	3.34	2.91
4.	15–19	7,305,219	3,122,258	4,182,961	3.57	1.53	2.04
5.	20–24	8,515,187	1,865,382	6,649,806	4.16	0.91	3.25
6.	25–44	62,578,261	17,060,685	45,517,576	30.57	8.34	22.24
7.	45–64	45,139,324	19,013,947	26,125,377	22.05	9.29	12.76
8.	65 & over	9,136,783	4,877,390	4,259,393	4.46	2.38	2.08
9.	Unknown	0	0	0	0.00	0.00	0.00
10.	Total	157,667,818	59,644,404	98,023,414	77.03	29.14	47.89

Schedule 4—Hospital Cost Analysis by Age and Gender
Hospital
All Regions

	A Age	B Total ($)	C Male ($)	D Female ($)	E Total PMPM($)	F Male PMPM($)	G Female PMPM($)
1.	Under 1	4,742,566	2,554,056	2,188,511	2.32	1.25	1.07
2.	1–4	1,239,990	766,817	473,173	0.61	0.37	0.23
3.	5–14	2,324,710	1,333,289	991,422	1.14	0.65	0.48
4.	15–19	1,810,959	727,851	1,083,100	0.88	0.36	0.53
5.	20–24	2,389,557	571,741	1,817,815	1.17	0.28	0.89
6.	25–44	16,523,659	4,580,113	11,943,546	8.07	2.24	5.84
7.	45–64	15,696,260	8,164,748	7,531,512	7.67	3.99	3.68
8.	65 & over	4,104,158	2,307,919	1,796,239	2.01	1.13	0.88
9.	Unknown	0	0	0	0.00	0.00	0.00
10.	Total	48,831,861	21,006,534	27,825,327	23.86	10.26	13.59
11.	Grand Total (schedules 3 and 4)	206,499,679	80,650,937	125,848,741	100.89	39.40	61.49

Schedule 5—Hospital Services

A Type of Services (Excluding Medicare)	B Number of Cases	C Total Inpatient Days Incurred	D Total Cost ($)	E Average Cost per Case ($)
1. General medical	4,030	20,686	14,760,467	3,662
2. Surgical	3,383	18,184	18,340,579	5,422
3. Obstetrical	2,878	8,340	5,694,952	1,979
4. Pediatric	1,101	4,058	2,996,473	2,721
5. Mental health	581	6,282	2,268,856	3,906
6. Newborn	2,636	8,109	3,342,149	1,268
7. Other	0	0	0	0
8. *Total*	14,609	65,659	47,403,475	3,245
9. C.O.B.	0	0	3,251,824	0
10. *Total*	14,609	65,659	50,655,299	3,467
11. Medicare	0	0	0	0
12. Medicaid	492	1,972	1,428,387	2,902
13. *Grand total*	15,101	67,631	52,083,686	3,449

A Comparison of Two Hospital Agreements with Managed Care Organizations

Hospital Agreement with "WORST" Health Plan

This Agreement is entered into on this first day of _____ by and between the World's Oldest Renowned Simply Terrific Health Plan, Inc. ("WORST Health Plan") and _____ Hospital ("Hospital"). Under this Agreement, Hospital becomes a member of WORST Health Plan's Provider Network, and both parties agree to abide by the terms and conditions contained in this Agreement.

I. Definitions

   A. *Copayments* are those amounts that a Member is required to pay to a provider at the time health services are rendered in accordance with the terms of a Subscriber Agreement.

   B. *Covered Services* means all inpatient, emergency, and outpatient services which are available at, and provided by, Hospital to a Member and for which a health benefit is provided to a Member pursuant to a Subscriber Agreement.

   C. *Deductible* is that amount that a member is required to pay to providers of health care services before becoming eligible for benefits in accordance with the terms of a Subscriber Agreement.

   D. *Member* means any person on whose behalf a Subscriber Agreement has been entered into with Health Plan for the provision of Covered Services.

   E. *Participating Physician* means a physician who has agreed in writing to provide Covered Services to Health Plan's Members, and to comply with the reimbursement mechanisms and utilization review and quality assurance programs established by Health Plan.

   F. *Payer* means an employer, trust fund, insurance carrier, health care service plan, or any other entity which has an obligation to provide certain medical services or benefits to a Member,

(WORST Health Plan Agreement continued on page 72)

Hospital Agreement with "GOOD" Health Plan

This Agreement is entered into on this first day of _____ by and between the Great Old Original Doctors Health Plan, Inc. ("GOOD Health Plan") and _____ Hospital ("Hospital"). Under this Agreement, Hospital becomes a member of GOOD Health Plan's Provider Network, and both parties agree to abide by the terms and conditions contained in this Agreement.

I. Definitions
   A. *Copayments* are those amounts that a Member is required to pay to a provider at the time health services are rendered in accordance with the terms of a Subscriber Agreement.

   B. *Covered Services* means all impatient, emergency, and out-patient services which are available at, and provided by, Hospital to a Member and for which a health benefit is provided to a Member *pursuant to the terms of the Products described in Attachment A. Covered Services shall not include any professional component of Hospital service, except with respect to those services specifically set forth in Attachment B.*

   C. *Deductible* is that amount that a member is required to pay to providers of health care services before becoming eligible for benefits in accordance with the terms of a Subscriber Agreement.

   D. *Member* means any person on whose behalf a Subscriber Agreement has been entered into with Health Plan for the provision of Covered Services, *as evidenced by a Member identification card.*

   E. *Participating Physician* means a physician who has agreed in writing to provide Covered Services to Health Plan's Members and to comply with the reimbursement mechanism and utilization review and quality assurance programs established by Health Plan.

(GOOD Health Plan Agreement continued on page 73)

(WORST Health Plan Agreement continued)

or any other entity which has contracted with Health Plan to use Hospital's services.

G. *Products* means the terms and conditions of, and health care services offered to Members pursuant to, a Subscriber Agreement.

H. *Subscriber Agreement* means the contract between Health Plan and a Payer, employer, individual, labor union, trust, association, partnership, or other group which specifies the health care services to be provided by Health Plan to Members enrolled in one of its Products, and the terms and conditions for the provision of such services.

II. Provision of Services

Hospital shall provide those Covered Services to Health Plan Members which it customarily provides to its other patients in accordance with applicable standards and procedures.

III. Compensation and Billing

A. Health Plan or Payer agrees to pay Hospital for all services rendered to Members according to the compensation schedule specified in Attachment A. Hospital agrees to accept this rate as payment in full.

B. Hospital shall submit all claims for Covered Services to Health Plan within 30 days of the date of a Member's discharge from Hospital or, in the case of outpatient services, 30 days after the services are rendered. Claims received after this 30-day period may be denied for payment. Hospital shall submit such claims in a billing format acceptable to Health Plan and Payer.

C. Hospital claims for emergency room services must include a copy of Member's emergency room summary sheet. Claims not containing this information may not be paid.

D. Health Plan or Payer will pay Hospital's claims for Covered Services when such claims are accurate, complete, and in the form designated in Section III-B of this Agreement.

(WORST Health Plan Agreement continued on page 74)

(GOOD Health Plan Agreement continued)

F. *Products* means the terms and conditions of, and health care services offered to Members pursuant to, a Subscriber Agreement.

G. *Subscriber Agreement* means the contract between Health Plan and an employer, individual, labor union, trust, association, partnership, or other group which specifies the health care services to be provided by Health Plan to Members enrolled in one of its Products, and the terms and conditions for the provision of such services.

II. Provision of Services
Hospital shall provide those Covered Services to Health Plan Members which it customarily provides to its other patients in accordance with applicable standards and procedures.

III. Compensation and Billing
A. Health Plan agrees to pay Hospital for Covered Services rendered to Members according to the compensation schedule specified in Attachment B.

B. Hospital shall submit all claims for Covered Services to Health Plan within 30 days of the date of Member's discharge from Hospital or, in the case of outpatient services, 30 days after the services are rendered, *or from the date of verification of a patient's status as a Member, whichever is latest. Hospital shall submit such claims on billing form UBF or a form containing equivalent information.*

C. Health Plan will pay Hospital's claims for Covered Services *within 30 days of receipt* when such claims are accurate, complete, and in the form designated in Section III-B of this Agreement.

(GOOD Health Plan Agreement continued on page 75)

E. Hospital agrees that payment by Health Plan or Payer in accordance with this Agreement constitutes payment in full for all services rendered to Members, and further agrees that in no event, including but not limited to nonpayment by Health Plan, Health Plan's insolvency, or breach of this Agreement, shall Hospital bill, charge, collect a deposit from, seek compensation from, remuneration from, or have any recourse against any Member(s) or other person acting on their behalf other than Health Plan for services provided pursuant to this Agreement. Hospital further agrees that: (1) this provision shall survive the termination of this Agreement regardless of the cause giving rise to termination and shall be construed to be for the benefit of Members; (2) this provision supersedes any oral or written contrary agreement now written or hereafter entered into between Hospital and any Member(s) or persons acting on their behalf; and (3) any modifications, additions, or deletions to the provisions of this Section III-E shall become effective on a date no earlier than fifteen (15) days after the New York Commissioner of Health has received notice of such proposed change.

F. However, neither Member nor Health Plan shall be liable for payment for any Covered Service which is determined in advance by Health Plan and communicated in writing to the Hospital to be medically unnecessary (except that Members shall be liable for medically unnecessary emergency room care as determined by Health Plan and confirmed by Health Plan's Grievance Procedure); provided however: if a Member requests health care services after being informed by Hospital prior to the rendering of such services that the services have been determined to be medically unnecessary by Health Plan, such Member shall be solely liable for payment. This Section III-F shall survive the termination of this Agreement and shall supersede any oral or written contrary agreement heretofore entered into between Hospital and any Member or persons acting on a Member's behalf.

G. Health Plan shall distribute an identification card to Members which Hospital shall rely on for determinations regarding eligibility status of members, unless notified of a Member's

(WORST Health Plan Agreement continued on page 76)

(GOOD Health Plan Agreement continued)

D. Hospital agrees that payment by Health Plan in accordance with the Agreement constitutes payment in full for services rendered to Members and further agrees that in no event, including but not limited to nonpayment by Health Plan, Health Plan's insolvency, or breach of this Agreement, shall Hospital bill, charge, collect a deposition form , seek compensation, remuneration from, or have any recourse against any Member(s) or other person acting on their behalf other than Health Plan for services provided pursuant to this Agreement. *Except as set forth in Section III-E, this provision shall not prohibit collection of deductibles, copayment, payment for noncovered services or payments described in Section III-G.* Hospitals further agrees that: (1) this provision shall survive the termination of this Agreement regardless of the cause giving rise to termination and shall be construed to be for the benefit of Members; (2) this provision supersedes any oral or written contrary agreement now written or hereafter entered into between Hospital and Member(s) or persons acting on their behalf; and (3) any modifications, additions, or deletions to the provisions of this Section III-D shall become effective on a date no earlier than fifteen (15) days after the New York Commissioner of Health has received notice of such proposed change.

E. However, neither Member nor Health Plan shall be liable for payment for any Covered Service which is determined in advance by Health Plan and communicated in writing to the Hospital to be medically unnecessary (except that Members shall be liable for medically unnecessary emergency room care as determined by Health Plan and confirmed by Health Plan's Grievance Procedure); provided however: if a Member requests health care services after being informed by Hospital prior to the rendering of such services that the services have been determined to be medically unnecessary by Health Plan, such Member shall be solely liable for payment. This Section III-E shall survive the termination of this Agreement and shall supersede any oral or written contrary agreement heretofore entered into between Hospital and any Member or persons acting on a Member's behalf.

F. Health Plan shall distribute an identification card to Members, which Hospital shall rely on for determinations regarding eligibility status of members, unless notified of a Member's

(GOOD Health Plan Agreement continued on page 77)

disenrollment, in which case Hospital shall be reimbursed for all Covered Services until the date of the Member's termination.

H. Hospital agrees to assist Health Plan and/or Payer to coordinate benefits with other third-party payers or third parties who are responsible for services rendered to Members. In any case where Member has coverage from any third party including Medicare and such third party is billed by Hospital for services also covered under Member's Subscriber Agreement, Health Plan or Payer will pay Hospital for services covered under Member's Group or individual Service Agreement that were not covered and paid by such other third party, subject to the provision that in no case will Health Plan or Payer pay Hospital an amount which would result in Hospital receiving more than one hundred percent of the amount required by this Agreement.

I. For Covered Services not available at Hospital during an inpatient stay, Hospital may, with prior approval of Health Plan, transport patient to another Participating Provider that provides such services. Hospital will bear the responsibility of paying such Participating Provider for any such Covered Service and for the appropriate transportation costs.

IV. Hospital Obligations

A. Hospital shall participate in and comply with the utilization management ("UM"), quality assurance ("QA"), and Member grievance ("MG") programs of Health Plan and Payers. These UM, QA, and MG policies and procedures may be amended from time to time. Any admission not in compliance with the UR program may be subject to retrospective denial for payment. In the event that Health Plan was unable to conduct or complete preadmission review or concurrent review prior to Member's discharge from Hospital, then Health Plan will conduct or complete such review after discharge.

B. Hospital shall maintain policies or professional liability insurance in an amount acceptable to Health Plan to insure Hospital, Health Plan, Payer, and their employees against claims arising under this Agreement. Documentary evidence of such insurance policy shall be provided to Health Plan.

(WORST Health Plan Agreement continued on page 78)

disenrollment, in which case Hospital shall be reimbursed for all Covered Services *until the date of notification.*

G. Hospital agrees to assist Health Plan to coordinate benefits with other third-party payers or third parties who are responsible for services rendered to Members. In any case where Member has coverage from any third party including Medicare and such third party is billed by Hospital for services also covered under Member's Subscriber Agreement, Health Plan will pay Hospital for services covered under Member's Group or individual Service Agreement that were not covered and paid by such other third party. *Nothing contained herein shall restrict or otherwise affect Hospital's rights or obligations with respect to compensation from other third-party payers at its regular rates.*

H. For Covered Services not available at Hospital, Hospital may, with prior approval of Health Plan, transport patient to another Provider that provides such services. *Health Plan agrees to pay such other Provider for this Covered Service and for transportation on an outpatient basis.*

IV. Hospital Obligations

A. Hospital shall participate in and comply with Health Plan's utilization management ("UM"), quality assurance ("QA"), and Member grievance ("MG") programs. *Copies of Health Plan's UM, QA, and MG policies and procedures are incorporated in this Agreement as Attachments C, D, and E respectively.*

B. Hospital shall maintain policies or professional liability insurance or a professional liability self-insurance plan *in the amount of at least $1 million per occurrence/$1 million aggregate and general liability to insure Hospital and its employees against claims arising under this Agreement.* Documentary evidence of such in-

(GOOD Health Plan Agreement continued on page 79)

C. Hospital represents and warrants that it is currently, and for the duration of this Agreement shall remain, (1) in full compliance with all applicable laws, including licensing laws; (2) accredited by the Joint Commission on Accreditation of Healthcare Organizations; and (3) in good standing under the Federal Medicare Program. Hospital shall provide Health Plan with a copy of its most recent JCAHO Accreditation report upon execution of this Agreement. Hospital shall provide Health Plan with copies of all future Accreditation reports and notices of failure to comply with federal, state, or local laws within five (5) working days of their receipt.

D. Hospital shall notify Health Plan within five (5) working days of the time that Hospital learns of the initiation of any action procedure or report against Hospital or any member of its staff, which might jeopardize Hospital's JCAHO Accreditation or which might impair Hospital's ability to perform its obligations under this Agreement.

E. Hospital shall notify Health Plan of any suits or claims filed against Hospital within five (5) working days of Hospital's receipt of notice of such claim having been filed. Hospital shall provide Health Plan with any information regarding such claims.

F. Hospital agrees that Health Plan may list Hospital in Health Plan's Participating Provider directory and may describe Hospital in Health Plan's marketing materials.

G. Hospital shall maintain medical records and billing records relating to Members for a time period sufficient to enable Health Plan and/or Payer to have access to such records for their purposes. Hospital shall allow appropriate Health Plan personnel direct and unlimited access to the hospital/medical records as necessary for utilization management and claims processing purposes

(WORST Health Plan Agreement continued on page 80)

surance policy *or policies or self-insurance plan shall be provided to Health Plan upon request, and Hospital shall provide notification to Health Plan of any material adverse change in coverage or its self-insurance plan within five (5) days of receiving notice of such change in coverage or self-insurance plan.*

C. Hospitals represents and warrants that it is currently, and for the duration of this Agreement shall remain, (1) in full compliance with all applicable laws, including licensing laws; (2) accredited by the Joint Commission on Accreditation of Healthcare Organizations; and (3) in good standing under the Federal Medicare Program. Hospitals shall provide *immediate notification to Health Plan of any actions to suspend, revoke, or restrict its license, accreditation, or Federal Medicare Program good standing.*

D. Hospital *agrees to make a good faith effort* to notify Health Plan *of the outcome of* any suits or claims filed against Hospital, by or relating to a Member, within five (5) working days of Hospital's receipt of notice *of such settlement. Subject to confidentiality restrictions,* Hospital shall provide Health Plan with any information regarding such claims reasonably requested by Health Plan.

E. Hospital agrees that Health Plan may list Hospital in Health Plan's Participating Provider directory and may describe Hospital in Health Plan's marketing materials. *All descriptive materials must be approved in advance by Hospital.*

F. Hospital shall maintain medical records and billing records relating to Members *and preserve them for such time periods as are required by applicable state and federal law, regulations, and practices. Such records shall be treated as confidential so as to comply with all state and federal laws and regulations regarding the confidentiality of patient records. Subject to such confidenti-*

(GOOD Health Plan Agreement continued on page 81)

and shall make copies of such records available to Health Plan and/or Payer at no cost. Hospital shall cooperate with Health Plan to facilitate the information and record exchanges required for quality management, utilization management, peer review, or other programs required for Health Plan's operations.

H. Hospital shall cooperate with Health Plan's procedures for administering its credentialing and recertification standards, which Health Plan retains sole discretion to establish and modify. Hospital shall, upon Health Plan's reasonable request, execute consents to the release to Health Plan of information regarding Hospital by the American Hospital Association, JCAHO, and/or other such organizations and/or professional liability carriers.

I. Hospital shall comply with all applicable requirements set forth in Health Plan's Administrative Manual and in other program materials furnished by Health Plan.

J. Hospital agrees that in all communications with and in all actions on behalf of Members, it shall take no actions or make any communications which could undermine the confidence of anyone in Health Plan's programs.

(WORST Health Plan Agreement continued on page 82)

(GOOD Health Plan Agreement continued)

ality requirements, Hospital shall make copies of such records reasonably available at a cost of $.25 per page to Health Plan representatives, employees, or designees; the New York State Department of Health; and any other federal or state regulatory agency authorized by law, during the term of this Agreement and as may be reasonably requested following termination. Further, Hospital agrees to comply with record-keeping and record inspection requirements of federal, state, or local government programs or contracts.

V. Health Plan Obligations

A. Health Plan agrees to provide Hospital with descriptions of all plans and copies of all Subscriber Agreements currently in force and being marketed by Health Plan. Health Plan further agrees to offer Hospital staff an orientation program to describe the benefits provided by the Health Plan's products and the procedures required to comply with Health Plan's policies.

B. Health Plan agrees to provide Hospital with the names and telephone numbers of Health Plan staff to be contacted in order to verify enrollment, dependent coverage, benefit level, and status of any coinsurance and/or deductibles.

C. Health Plan agrees to provide Hospital with copies of its annual audit, quarterly and annual report filings to the New York State Division of Insurance, and any rate increase and new product applications. Health Plan further agrees to immediately notify Hospital if its status as an Article 44 HMO changes in any way and/or if any change is made in its rating by a reputable

(GOOD Health Plan Agreement continued on page 83)

(WORST Health Plan Agreement continued)

V. Term and Termination

A. The term of this Agreement shall commence on the date first written above, shall continue in effect for a period of one year, and shall automatically renew for one-year terms under the same terms and conditions, unless terminated pursuant to this Section.

B. Health Plan may terminate this Agreement without cause by giving Hospital 30 days' notice.

C. Health Plan may suspend this Agreement at any time for quality assurance concerns.

(WORST Health Plan Agreement continued on page 84)

(GOOD Health Plan Agreement continued)

Rating Agency (that is, A. M. Best, Moody's, Standard & Poors, and so forth).

D. *Health Plan shall maintain policies or professional liability insurance or a professional liability self-insurance plan in the amount of at least $1 million per occurrence/$1 million aggregate and general liability and such other insurance as shall be necessary to insure Health Plan and its employees against any other claim or claims for damages arising under this Agreement. Documentary evidence of such insurance shall be provided to Hospital. Health Plan shall notify hospital of any adverse change in this insurance coverage.*

VI. Term and Termination

A. The term of this Agreement shall commence on the date first written above, shall continue in effect for a period of one year, and, *with the exception of financial terms as per Attachment B*, shall automatically renew for one-year terms, unless terminated pursuant to this Section.

B. *This Agreement may be terminated without cause on the initial renewal date of the Agreement or at any time thereafter by either party giving the other party 90 days' notice. In the event either party materially breaches this Agreement, and the other party gives notice specifying the breach, both parties shall confer in good faith to resolve any dispute relating to the breach. If within 30 days of the notice such dispute remains unresolved and the breach is not cured, this Agreement may be terminated immediately by notice to the breaching party. This Agreement may be terminated immediately by either party without notice in the event the other party's license is revoked.*

C. Health Plan may suspend this Agreement *upon written notice to Hospital if quality assurance concerns meet the criteria identified in Health Plan's quality assurance program for such suspension (Attachment D). If after given the opportunity to remedy the issue(s) identified within 30 days of such written notice the Hospital fails to do so, this Agreement shall automatically terminate.*

(GOOD Health Plan Agreement continued on page 85)

(WORST Health Plan Agreement continued)

D. Following any termination of this Agreement by Health Plan, Hospital agrees to continue to provide Covered Services to Health Plan Members for 180 days at the rates agreed to under this Agreement.

E. In the event a Member is under treatment in Hospital at the time the obligations described in this Agreement terminate, Hospital and Health Plan shall continue to abide by the terms of this Agreement for that Member. In the event of Health Plan's insolvency, Hospital will continue to provide Covered Services to Members until the date of discharge. Hospital shall not, under any circumstances, bill Members for Covered Services rendered during this period.

VI.   Miscellaneous

A. Hospital agrees to indemnify, defend, and hold harmless Health Plan and/or Payer from any claim, real or imaginary, suit, cost, or expense incurred by Health Plan or Payer as a result of the actions of Hospital or its employees in connection with the performance of the terms and conditions of this Agreement.

B. None of the provisions of this Agreement or Health Plan's program are intended to create, nor shall be deemed or construed to create, any relationship between Health Plan and Hospital other than that of independent entities contracting with each other solely for the purpose of effecting the provisions of this Agreement and

(WORST Health Plan Agreement continued on page 86)

(GOOD Health Plan Agreement continued)

D. Upon suspension of either party's license or insurance coverage, either party may suspend this Agreement by giving written notice to the other party. If license or insurance coverage is not reinstated within 30 days of such notice, this Agreement shall automatically terminate.

E. Following any termination of this Agreement by Health Plan, Hospital agrees to continue to provide Covered Services to Health Plan Members *at its regular reimbursement rates.*

F. In the event a Member is under treatment in Hospital at the time the obligations described in this Agreement terminate, Hospital and Health Plan shall continue to abide by the terms of this Agreement for that Member *until such Member is transferred to another participating hospital or until treatment is completed.* In the event of Health Plan's insolvency, Hospital will continue to provide Covered Services to Members until the date of discharge. *With the exception of copayments and deductibles,* Hospital shall not, under any circumstances, bill Members for Covered Services rendered during this period.

VII. Miscellaneous
    A. Neither party shall utilize any trade name or service mark of the other party, or any material or property protected by patents, trademarks, or copyrights of the other party, except as expressly permitted by this Agreement or otherwise in writing.

B. *Hospital and Health Plan each agree to indemnify, defend, and hold harmless the other party* from any claim, real or imaginary, suit, cost, or expense incurred *by the other party* as a result of the actions *of the first party* or its employees in connection with the performance of the terms and conditions of this Agreement.

C. None of the provisions of this Agreement or Health Plan's program are intended to create, nor shall be deemed or construed to create, any relationship between Health Plan and Hospital other than that of independent entities contracting with each other solely for the purpose of effecting the provisions of this Agreement and of Health Plan's program. Neither Health Plan nor Hospital, nor

(GOOD Health Plan Agreement continued on page 87)

of Health Plan's program. Neither Health Plan nor Hospital, nor any of their respective employees, shall be construed to be the agent, employer, or representative of the other party.

C. Nothing in this Agreement shall be deemed to change or alter any relationship which exists or may come to exist between Hospital and any Member, and Health Plan shall not have the right to interfere with the care or treatment given or prescribed to any Member beyond Health Plan's UM program. Hospital shall have and be subject to the same duties, liabilities, and responsibilities toward Members as exist generally between patients and Hospital.

D. This Agreement may be amended by Health Plan by giving Hospital 30 days' prior written notice.

E. This Agreement, being intended to secure the services of Hospital, shall not be assigned, subcontracted, delegated, or transferred by Hospital without the prior written consent of Health Plan, and any attempted assignment, subcontract, delegation, or transfer shall be void. Health Plan may assign, subcontract, delegate, or transfer this Agreement without the prior written consent of Hospital.

F. Any notice required to be given pursuant to the terms and provisions of this Agreement shall be in writing and shall be sent via certified or registered mail, return receipt requested, postage prepaid, by prepaid express mail, or by hand delivery to the parties

(WORST Health Plan Agreement continued on page 88)

any of their respective employees, shall be construed to be the agent, employer, or representative of the other party.

D. Nothing in this Agreement shall be deemed to change or alter any relationship which exists or may come to exist between Hospital and any Member, and Health Plan shall not have the right to interfere with the care or treatment given or prescribed to any Member beyond *the UM program referred to in Section IV-A of this Agreement.* Hospital shall have and be subject to the same duties, liabilities, and responsibilities toward Members as exist generally between patients and Hospital.

E. This Agreement may be amended *only by mutual agreement in writing executed by the parties, except that this Agreement may be amended (1) by Health Plan to comply with applicable federal, state, or local laws or regulations; or (2) by Health Plan, by giving 60 days' prior written notice to Hospital of a proposed amendment, and such amendment shall be effective unless Hospital objects thereto in writing within 30 days of receiving such notice. Anything to the contrary contained herein notwithstanding, any amendment hereto must be approved in advance by the New York Commissioner of Health.*

F. This Agreement, being intended to secure the services of Hospital, shall not be assigned, subcontracted, delegated, or transferred by Hospital without the prior written consent of Health Plan, and any attempted assignment, subcontract, delegation, or transfer shall be void. *Health Plan may not assign, subcontract, delegate, or transfer this Agreement without the prior written consent of Hospital, except that Health Plan may assign this Agreement to any entity that controls, is controlled by, or is under common control with Health Plan now or in the future or which succeeds to its business as a result of a sale, merger, or other corporate transaction. Such Assignment requires prior notice to the New York State Department of Health and Division of Insurance.*

G. Any notice required to be given pursuant to the terms and provisions of the Agreement shall be in writing and shall be sent via certified or registered mail, return receipt requested, postage prepaid, by prepaid express mail, or by hand delivery to the parties at the addresses set forth on the signature page hereof.

(GOOD Health Plan Agreement continued on page 89)

at the addresses set forth on the signature page hereof.

G. This Agreement shall be construed in accordance with the laws of the State of New York. The invalidity or unenforceability of any terms or provisions hereof shall in no way affect the validity or enforceability of any other terms or provisions.

In witness whereof, the parties have executed this Agreement to be effective as of the date first written above.

By: _____   By: _____
Title: _____   Title: _____
Print name: _____   Print name: _____
Date: _____   Date: _____

(GOOD Health Plan Agreement continued)

H. This Agreement shall be construed in accordance with the laws of the State of New York. The invalidity of unenforceability of any terms or provisions hereof shall in no way affect the validity or enforceability of any other terms or provisions.

In witness whereof, the parties have executed this Agreement to be effective as of the date first written above.

By: _____   By: _____

Title: _____   Title: _____

Print name: _____   Print name: _____

Date: _____   Date: _____

Additional Books of Interest

Calculated Risk: A Provider's Guide to Assessing and Controlling the Financial Risk of Managed Care

edited by Bruce S. Pyenson, FSA, MAAA
Milliman & Robertson, Inc.

Calculated Risk presents the strategies and tools to help you analyze your current business and determine what needs to change to assume the various forms of managed care risk, including capitation. You'll benefit from experience-tested approaches, including the applications of actuarial cost models from the nation's foremost actuarial and consulting firm, Milliman & Robertson, Inc. The book is written in plain, easy-to-understand language and in a concise, executive-style format. For readers who want to explore topics more deeply or who want help in locating sources of data, the book concludes with a bibliography of additional resources.

Catalog No. E99-131001 (must be included when ordering)
1995. 80 pages, 19 figures, bibliography.
$32.00 (AHA members, $25.00)

Assessing Organizational Readiness for Capitation

edited by Deborah S. Kolb, PhD
Jennings Ryan & Kolb, Inc.

This innovative and highly user-friendly book from a leading management consulting firm provides a survey instrument that you can use to determine your institution's readiness for a capitated market and set organizationwide priorities that will help prepare for capitation and balance the needs of all stakeholders. This tool identifies your organization's critical needs along two dimensions: structural readiness and information readiness. Included with the survey instrument is an Organizational Readiness Matrix that helps you visualize whether your organization is well-positioned for capitation and, if it is not, where efforts should be focused to achieve a strong position.

Catalog No. F13-131002 (must be included when ordering)
1996. 90 pages, 8 figures, 7 tables.
$32.50 (AHA members, $26.00)

To order, call TOLL FREE 800-AHA-2626